WELLNESS JOURNAL

This journal belongs to

From

_____

To

_____

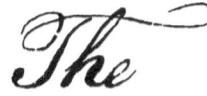

WELLNESS JOURNAL

SECOND EDITION

Robin Willis

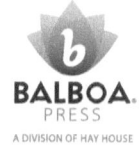

BALBOA.
PRESS

A DIVISION OF HAY HOUSE

Balboa Press books may be ordered through booksellers or by contacting:

Balboa Press
A Division of Hay House
1663 Liberty Drive
Bloomington, IN 47403
www.balboapress.com
1 (877) 407-4847

Because of the dynamic nature of the Internet, any web addresses or
links contained in this book may have changed since publication and may
no longer be valid. The views expressed in this work are solely those
of the author and do not necessarily reflect the views of the publisher,
and the publisher hereby disclaims any responsibility for them.

The author of this book does not dispense medical advice or prescribe the use
of any technique as a form of treatment for physical, emotional, or medical
problems without the advice of a physician, either directly or indirectly. The
intent of the author is only to offer information of a general nature to help
you in your quest for emotional and spiritual well-being. In the event you use
any of the information in this book for yourself, which is your constitutional
right, the author and the publisher assume no responsibility for your actions.

Any people depicted in stock imagery provided by Thinkstock are models,
and such images are being used for illustrative purposes only.
Certain stock imagery © Thinkstock.

Print information available on the last page.

ISBN: 978-1-5043-6312-9 (sc)
ISBN: 978-1-5043-6332-7 (e)

Balboa Press rev. date: 07/28/2016

I use the symbol of lavender throughout this Journal as a representation of its many healing properties. Lavender can heal skin disorders and insomnia, speeds up wound healing, has a calming effect as a tea, and used as a tonic for hair growth.

The sweet essence of lavender can create calmness, tranquility, and psychological well-being.

Be Calm
Stay Calm

ACKNOWLEDGEMENT

The idea that inspired and led me to write this Journal began as a desire to organize my medical information as well as my mother's medical history. The need to be my own doctor first shaped my thoughts in preparation for family doctor appointments, hospitalization, and other medical issues.

Ayanna Winslow, my sincere appreciation with your assistance in editing.

Thank you to all who supported this project, shared an insight, gave a suggestion, and provided your love. I'm forever grateful.

Charles Austin - much appreciation and gratefulness for all of your unending support, creative spirit, and medical contribution.

HOW TO USE THE WELLNESS JOURNAL

The second edition of The Wellness Journal continues to provide a way of maintaining medical information. Use it to keep all your medical records organized and to use as an inspirational journal. Inspirational and encouraging statements fill the Wellness Journal to support and assist you with charting your health information, emotions, and any issues or concerns.

You will find that when using the Journal your medical history will begin to tell a story and you will be in better control of your health. You will be more organized and clear about your medical history as you continue to update it.

It just takes one step to begin posting information in the Journal. It is that simple.

The Wellness Journal was born during my mother's illness with cancer. I needed a place to organize the enormous amount of information that we received during the first month of my mother's diagnosis. I began to write notes to myself. I used yellow sticky notes or I would tear pieces of paper to write down a thought or an important comment made by the nurse or someone in my mother's support group. One day, I noticed I had accumulated so many pieces of paper, sticky notes, and side notes on magazines that it was becoming difficult to keep up with. I brought a tablet and began writing and organizing the information and my thoughts. There were many notes regarding medication changes such as new and increased medications. There were various exams, specialty information, blood work, and more. I needed a place to organize it all. Moreover, it gave me a place to release my anxiety and sadness throughout her illness. Later, I valued the note taking and spending time to write important medical facts.

Years later, a diagnosis of thyroid disease challenged me. I needed a place of comfort to write down my thoughts, organize my health information, and to maintain my medical information. This was the beginning of the Wellness Journal. Using a journal made sense for me. It was very easy and it gave me control and another way of connecting with my healing by being in charge of my health and being my own doctor first.

Research states that record keeping and organizing information is difficult for the average person. The power to be in control of one's own story is an important factor when on a healing journey or finding a healthier lifestyle for oneself. The Wellness Journal will assist you preparing when you consult with your doctor or primary care provider. It will benefit you to spend time writing and posting information in your Wellness Journal to share with your primary care provider.

As you begin to use your Journal, it will serve as a support, a comfort, and a place for you to connect with your story. You will begin to view your personal medical information without judgmental statements or critical attitudes. It is your personal information.

Be in control of your medical story.
It's awesome! Try it.

Be Joy!

HOW PEOPLE HAVE USED THIS JOURNAL

This Journal really assisted my family and me through our journey of a recent illness. The inspiration notes and the space to write and reflect was just what I needed to stay organized and grounded. Anyone seeking a tool to use as an anchor...this book is it.
Annette Scruggs, MSA

The Wellness Journal Second Edition is a wonderful tool to keep track of your wellness journey. Robin Willis has created a necessary document to assist us in taking control of our health needs.
Ayana Mayes-Winslow, Educator

The previous Wellness Journal provided me with a vehicle in which to record all of my medications and medical concerns. I especially like the ability to take it to my doctor's office and have all of the information at my fingertips. I would certainly recommend this journal to everyone.
Christine Willis-Bennett, Montessori Teacher

CONTENTS

JOURNALING

Your Personal Story Begins

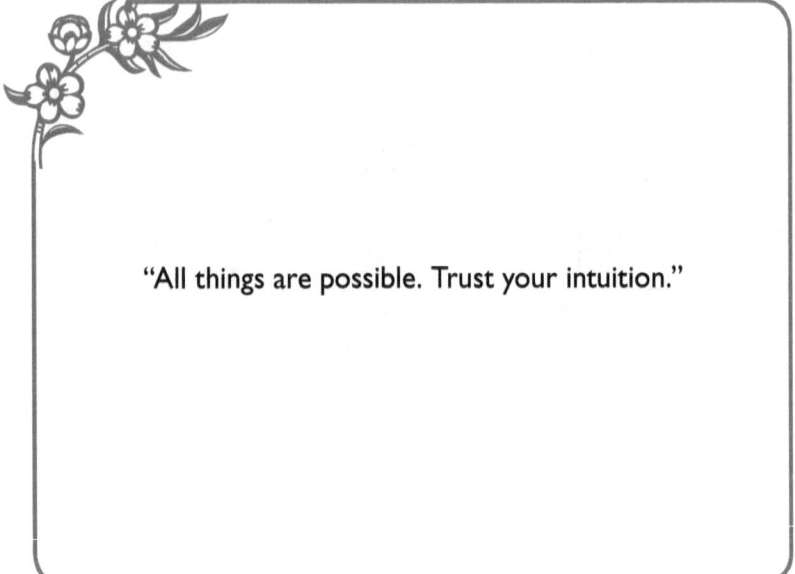

"All things are possible. Trust your intuition."

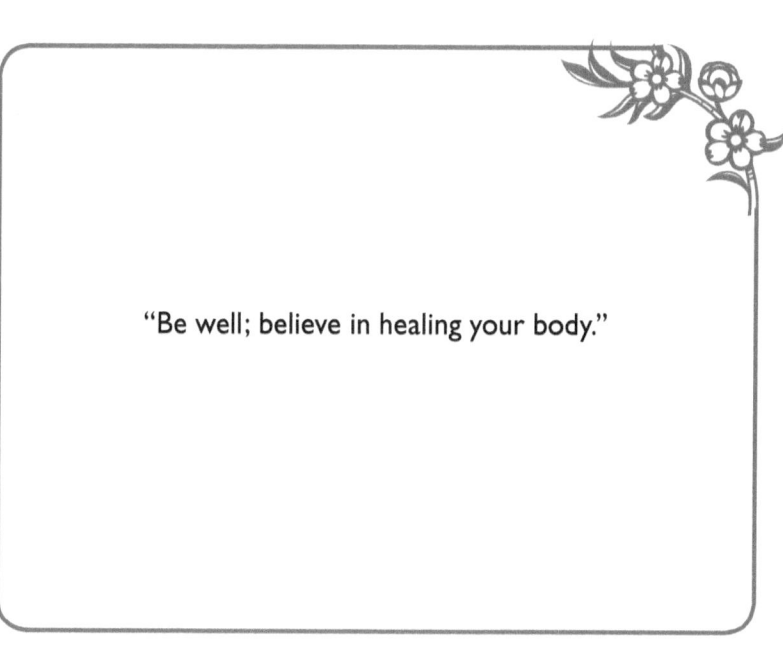

"Be well; believe in healing your body."

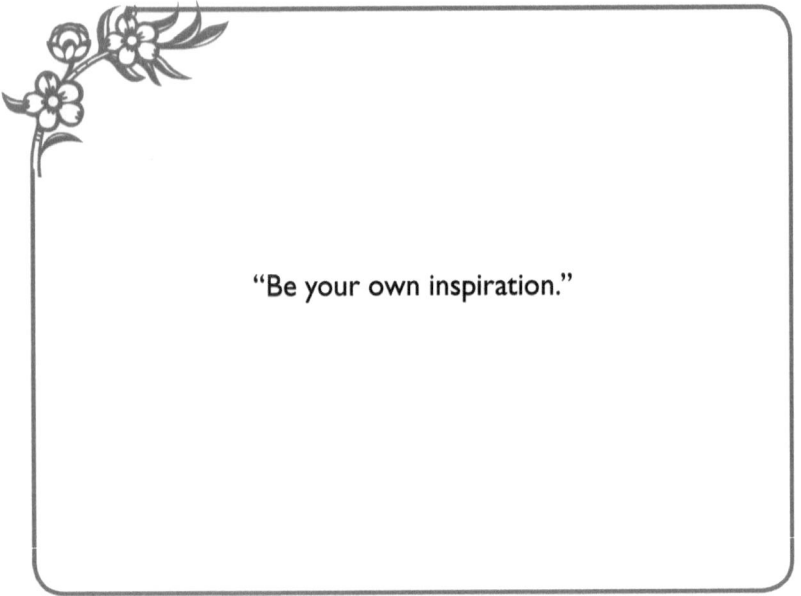

"Be your own inspiration."

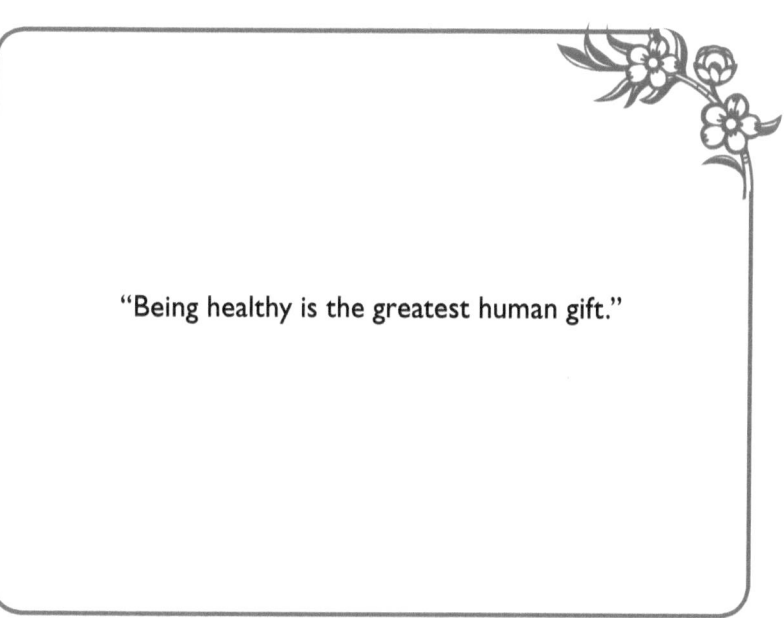

"Being healthy is the greatest human gift."

"Believe that the impossible is possible."
Jack & Cornelia Addington

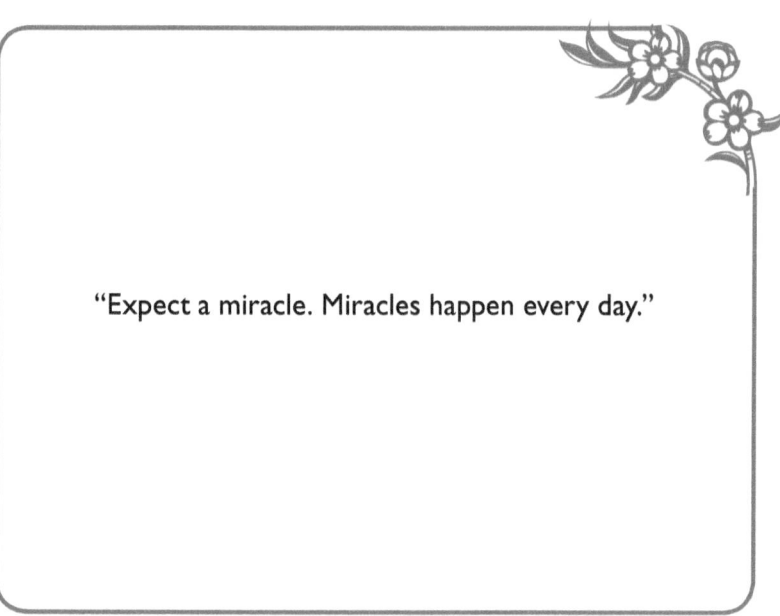

"Expect a miracle. Miracles happen every day."

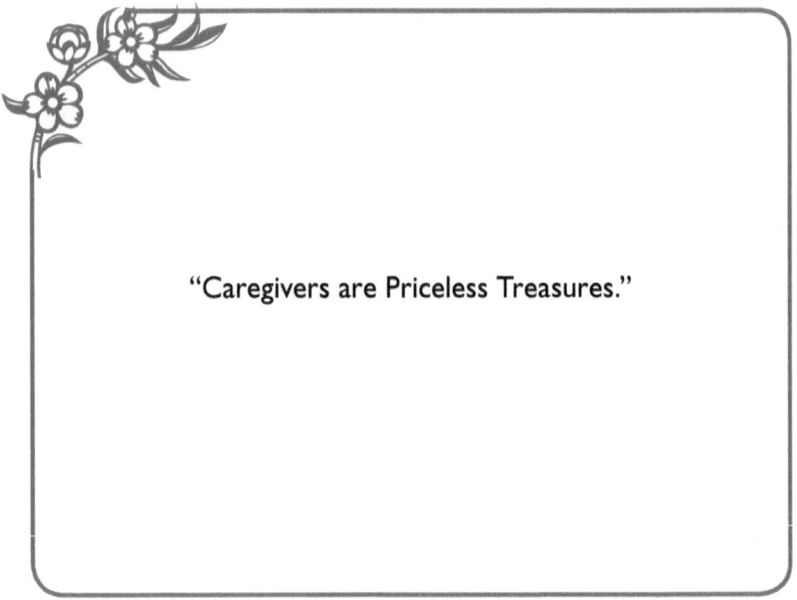

"Caregivers are Priceless Treasures."

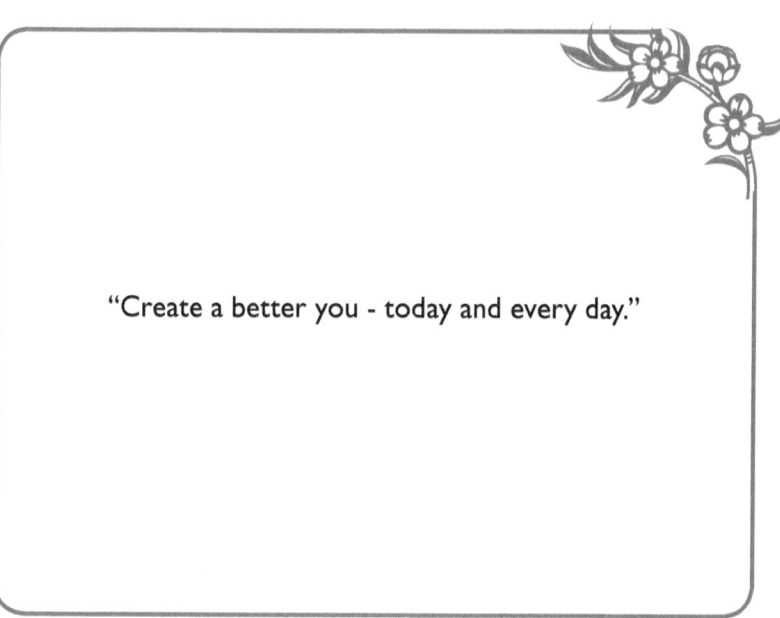

"Create a better you - today and every day."

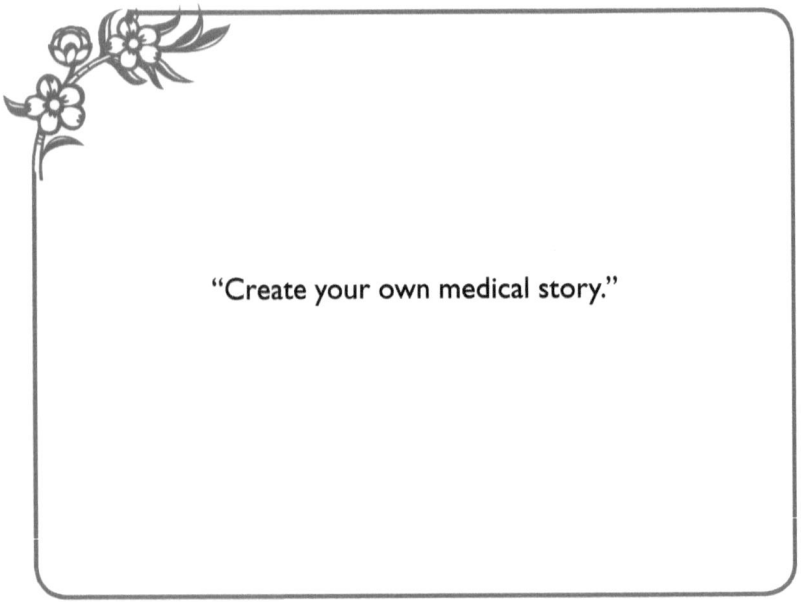

"Create your own medical story."

"Disability is not the hard winter of life.
It's just a situation."
Scott Whitaker, N.D. & Jose Fleming, CN, MH

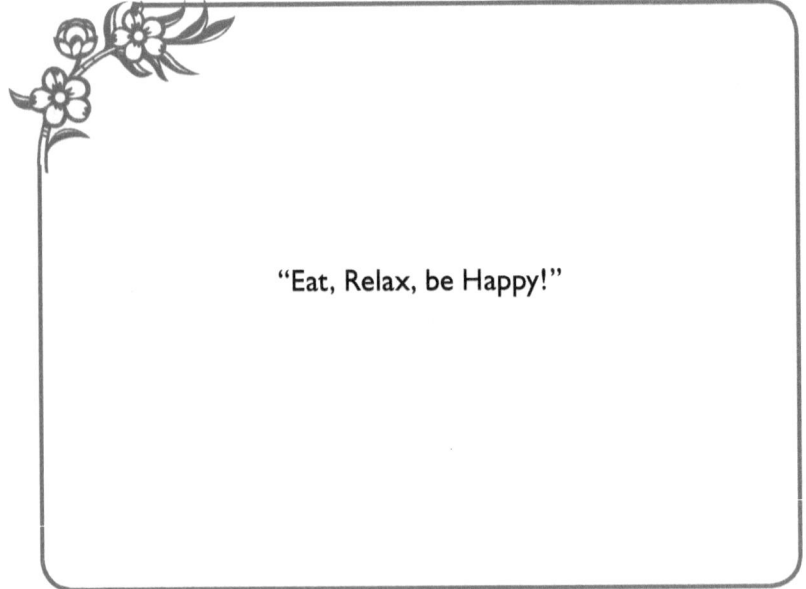

"Eat, Relax, be Happy!"

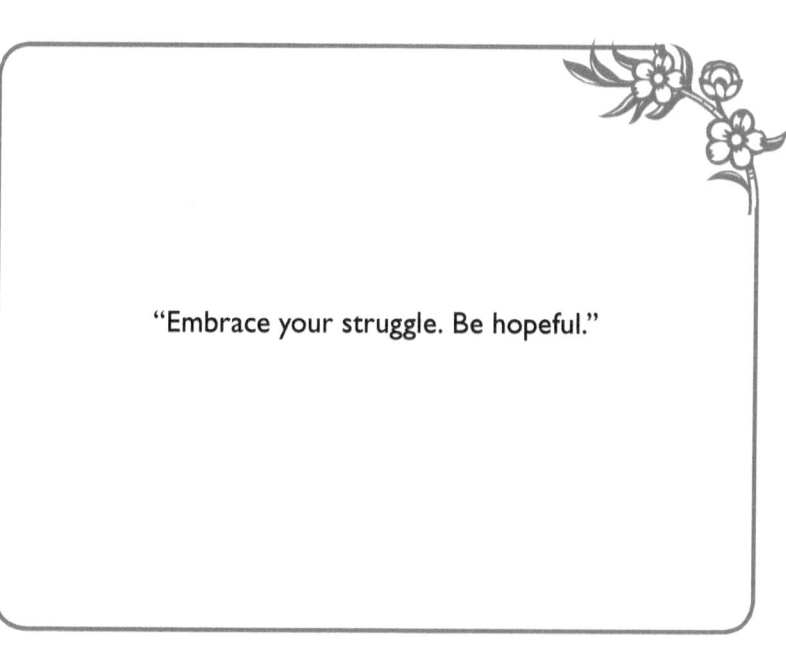

"Embrace your struggle. Be hopeful."

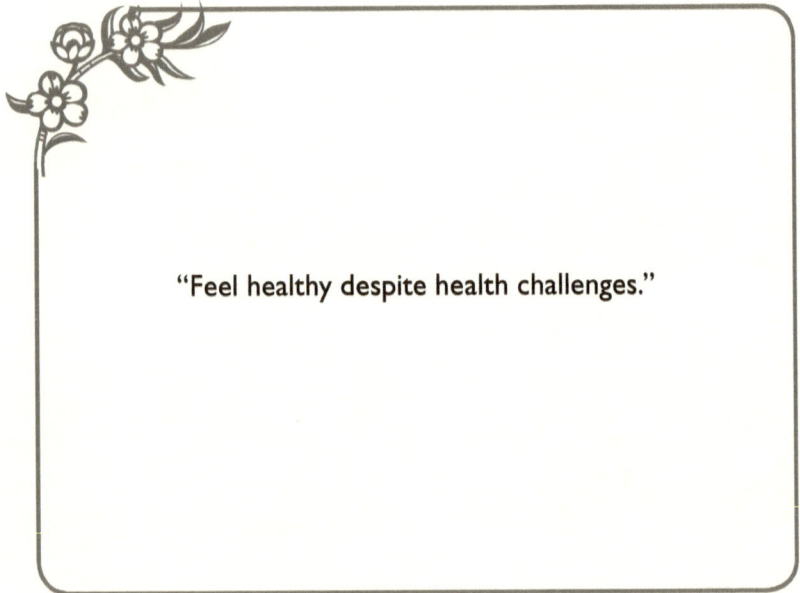

"Feel healthy despite health challenges."

"Give the gift of life, donate your organs."
American Organ Transplant Association

"God's will for you is perfect health."
Jack & Cornelia Addington

"Have a good night's sleep.
It can be better than gold."

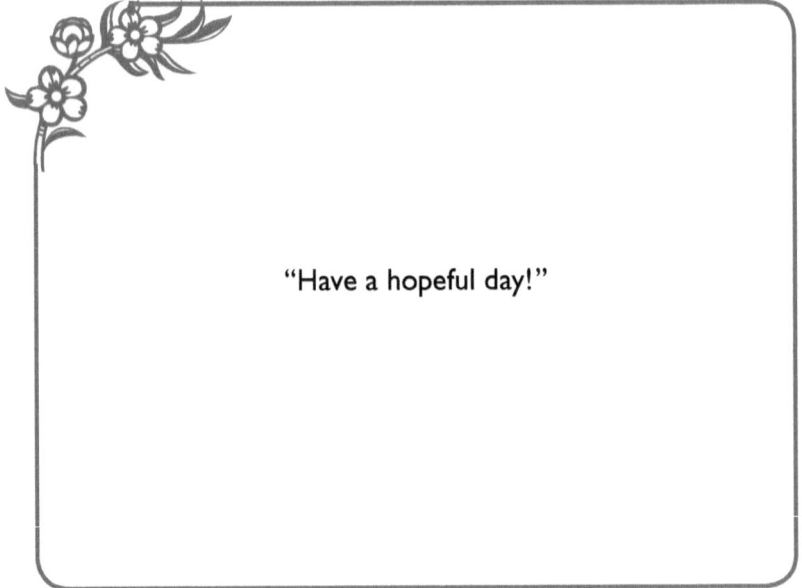

"Have a hopeful day!"

"Healing is a process.
It begins with acceptance from you."
Scott Whitaker, ND & Jose Fleming, CN,MH

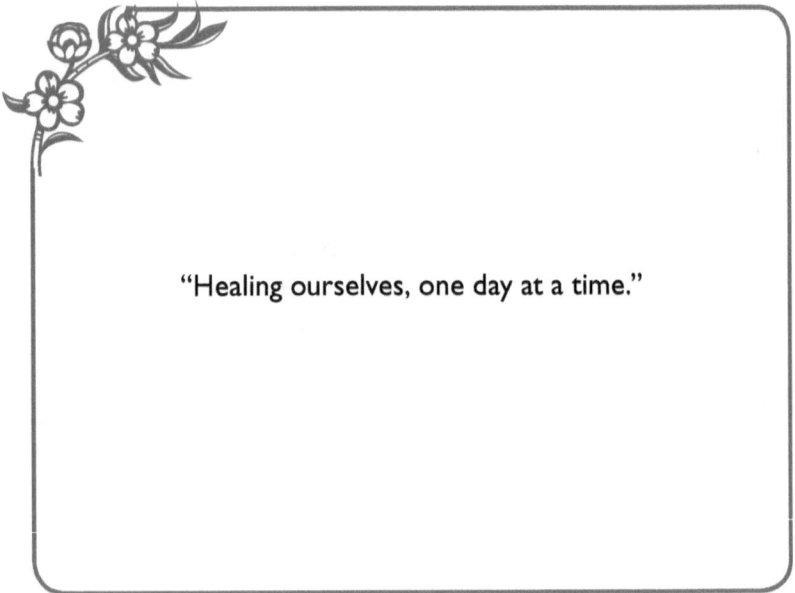

"Healing ourselves, one day at a time."

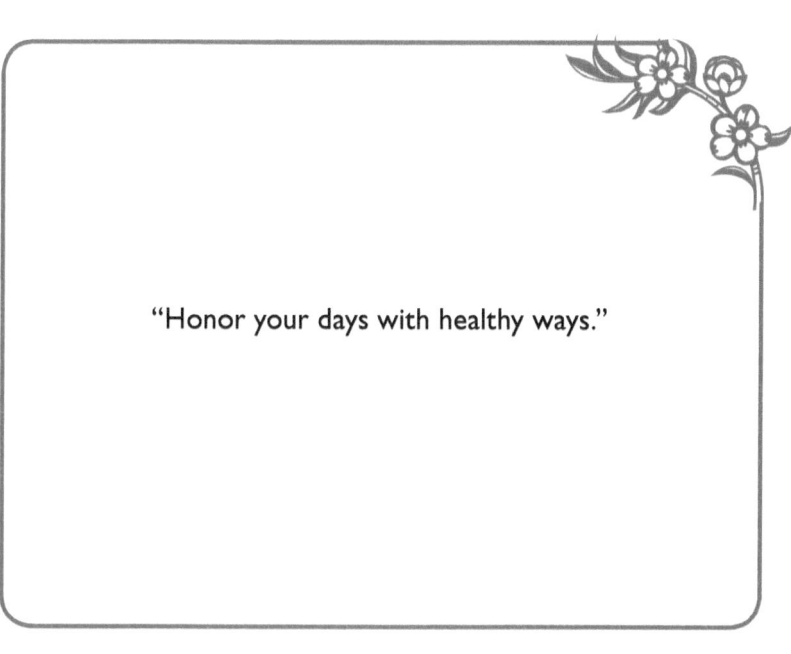

"Honor your days with healthy ways."

"Hope for today and live for all the tomorrows."
Rosemary Gladstar

"I have a disease, but the
disease does not have me."
William Sears M.D.

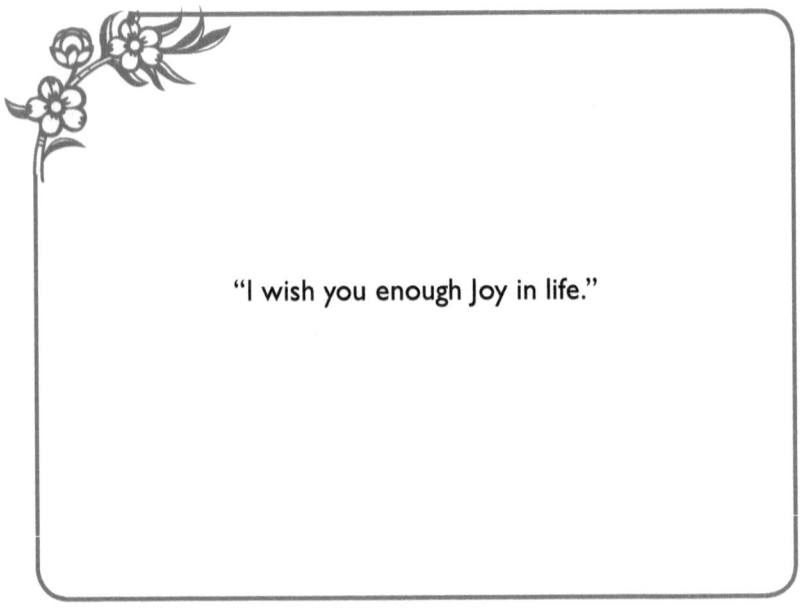

"I wish you enough Joy in life."

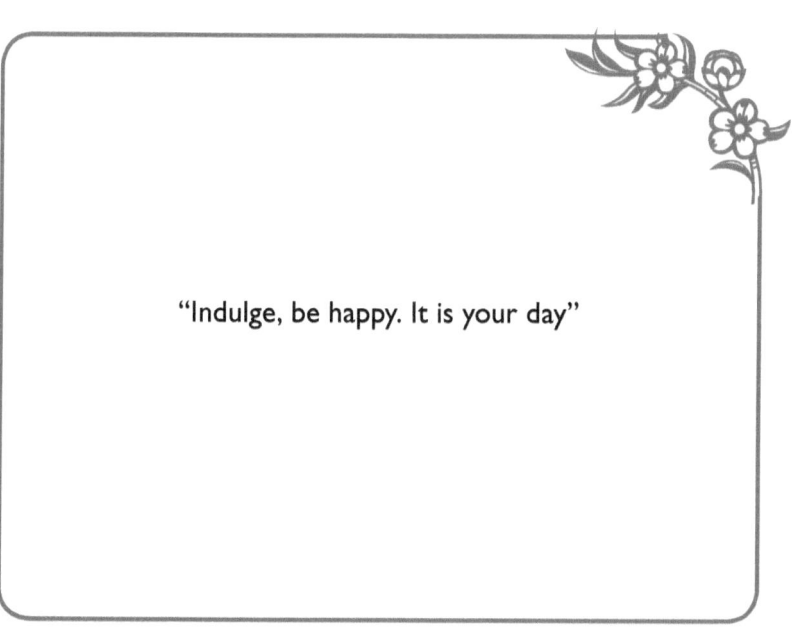

"Indulge, be happy. It is your day"

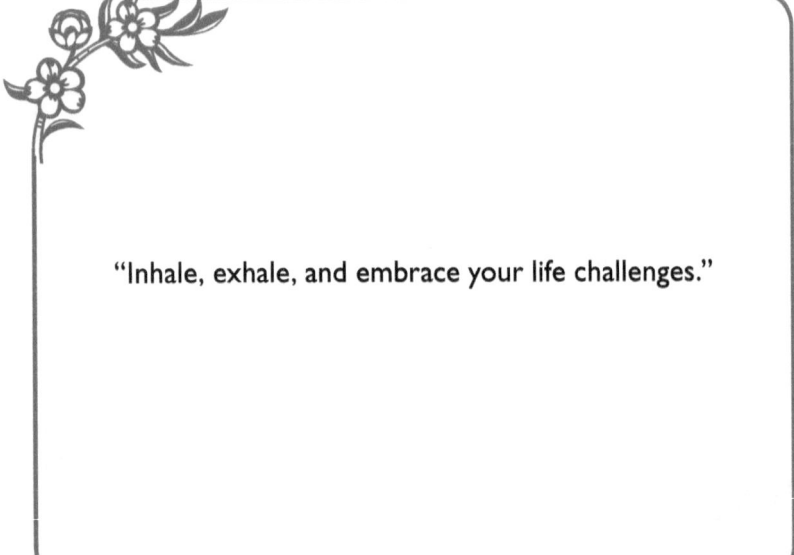

"Inhale, exhale, and embrace your life challenges."

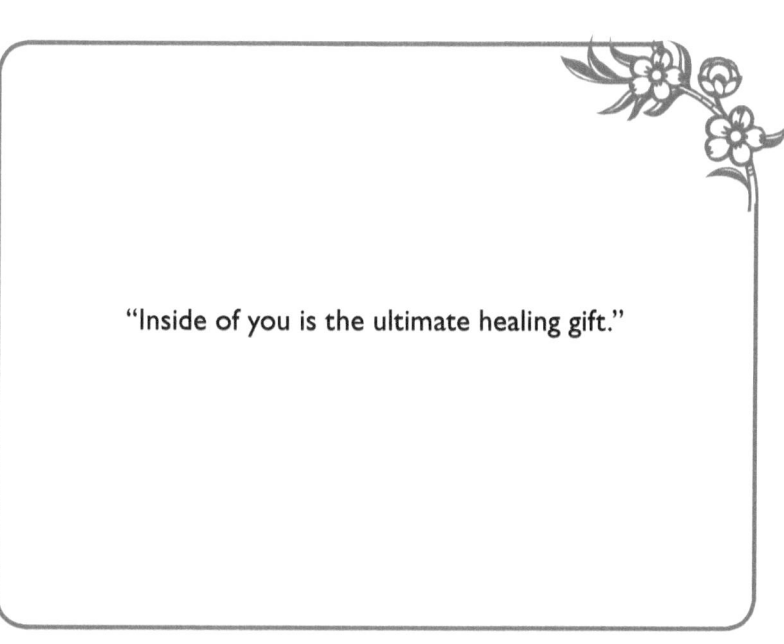

"Inside of you is the ultimate healing gift."

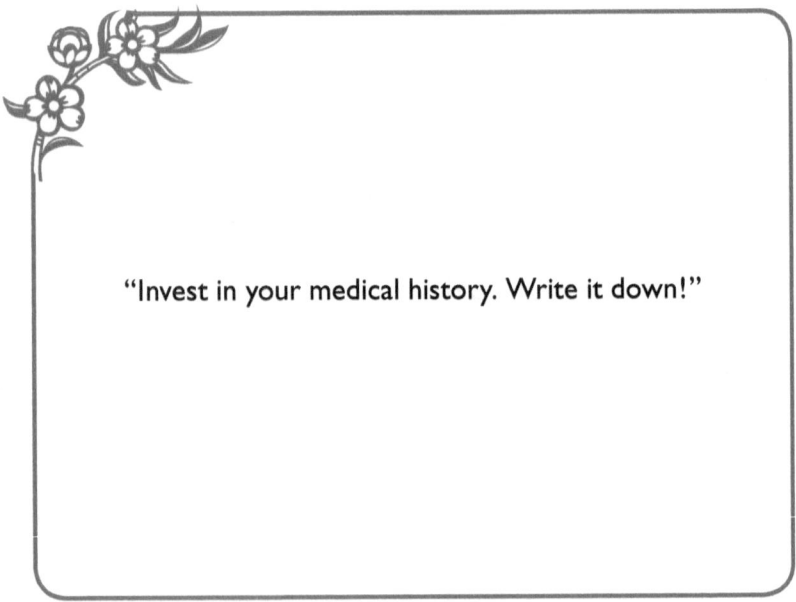

"Invest in your medical history. Write it down!"

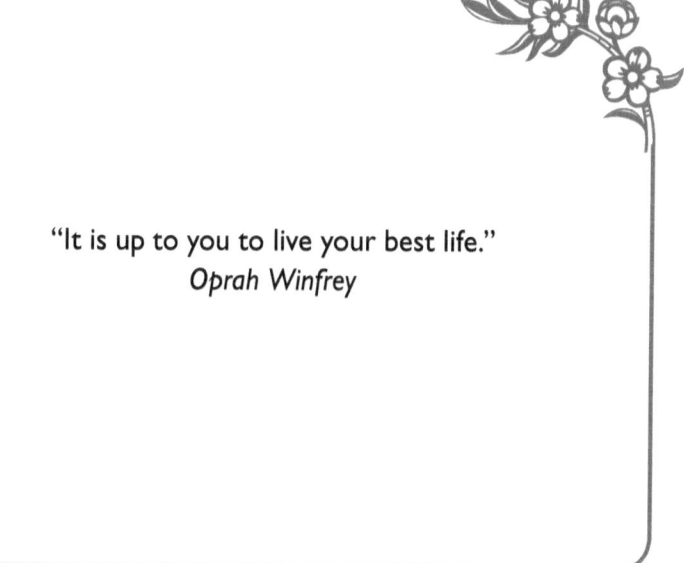

"It is up to you to live your best life."
Oprah Winfrey

"It's so healing to have an open and loving heart."

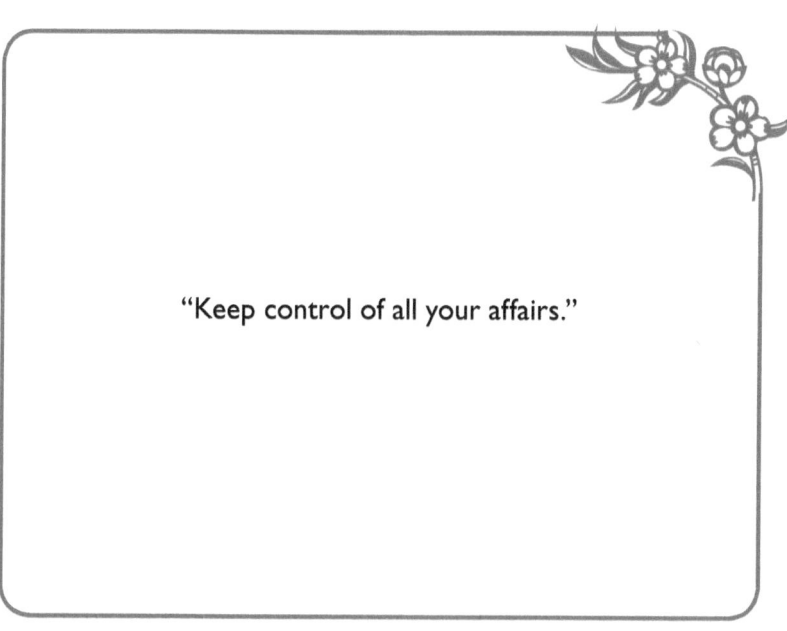

"Keep control of all your affairs."

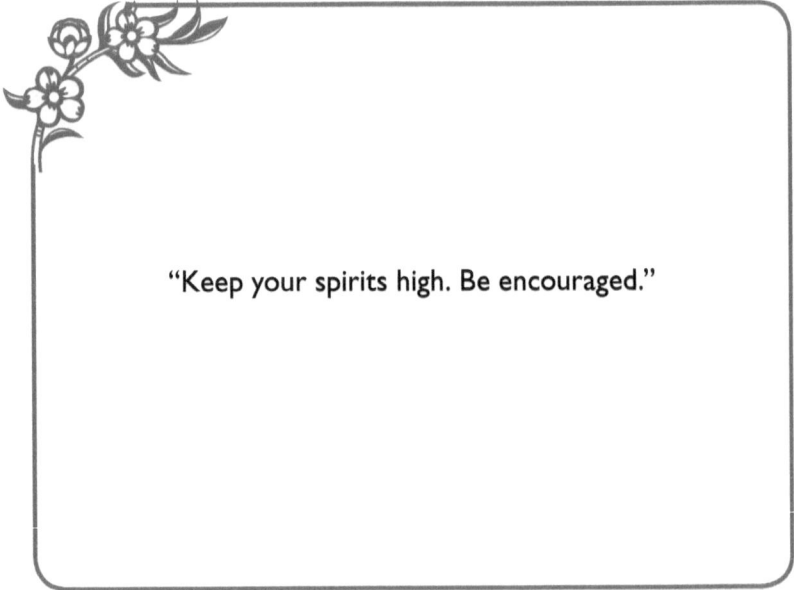

"Keep your spirits high. Be encouraged."

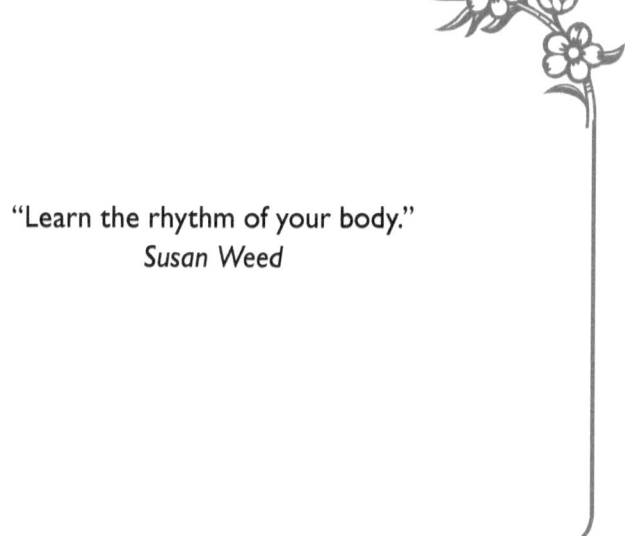

"Learn the rhythm of your body."
Susan Weed

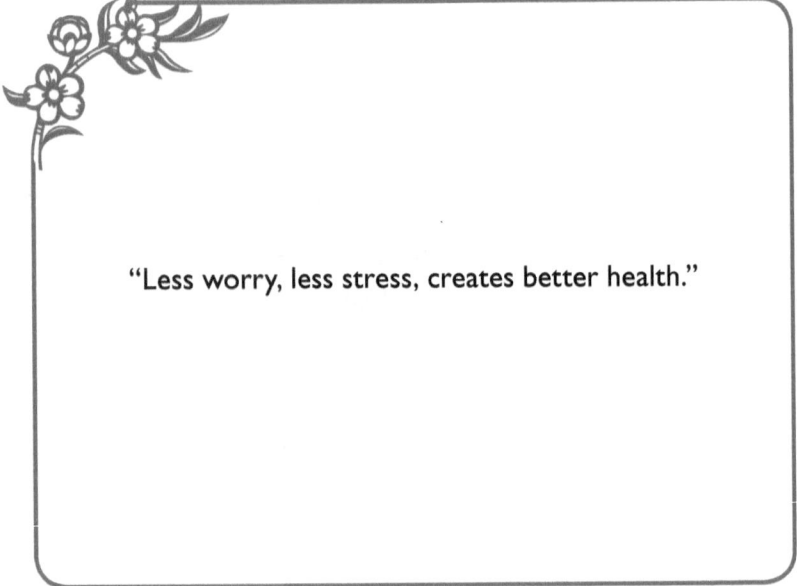

"Less worry, less stress, creates better health."

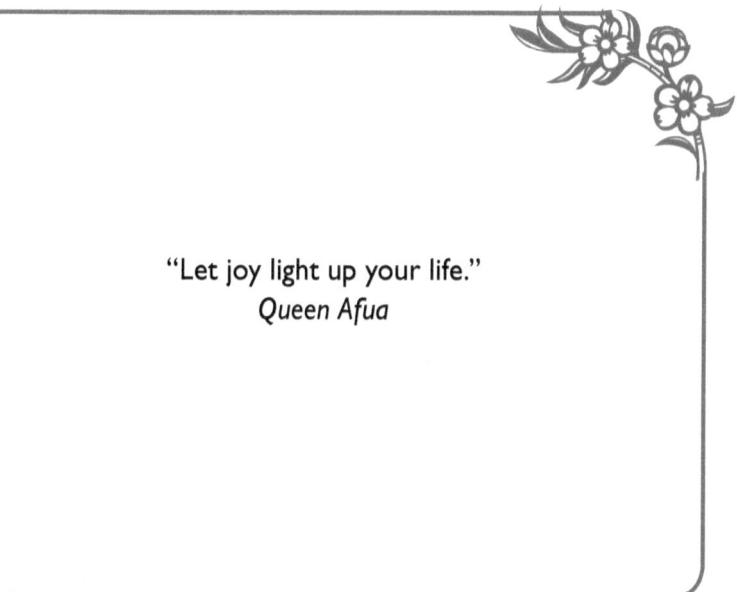

"Let joy light up your life."
Queen Afua

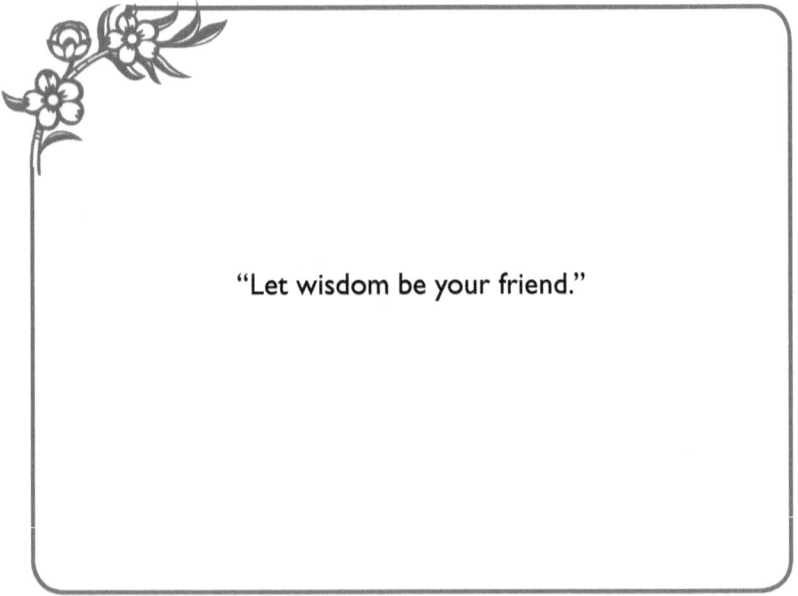

"Let wisdom be your friend."

"Celebrate yourself! Take long baths,
listen to great music, and be still."

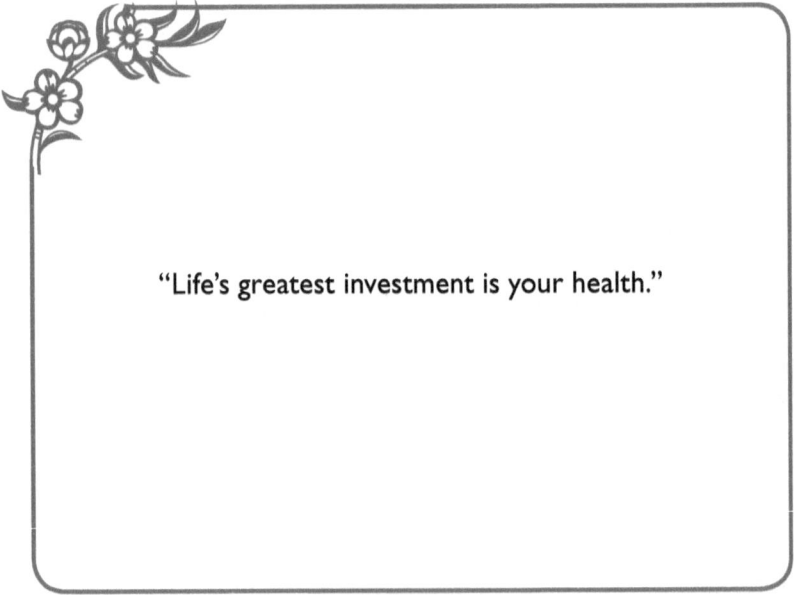

"Life's greatest investment is your health."

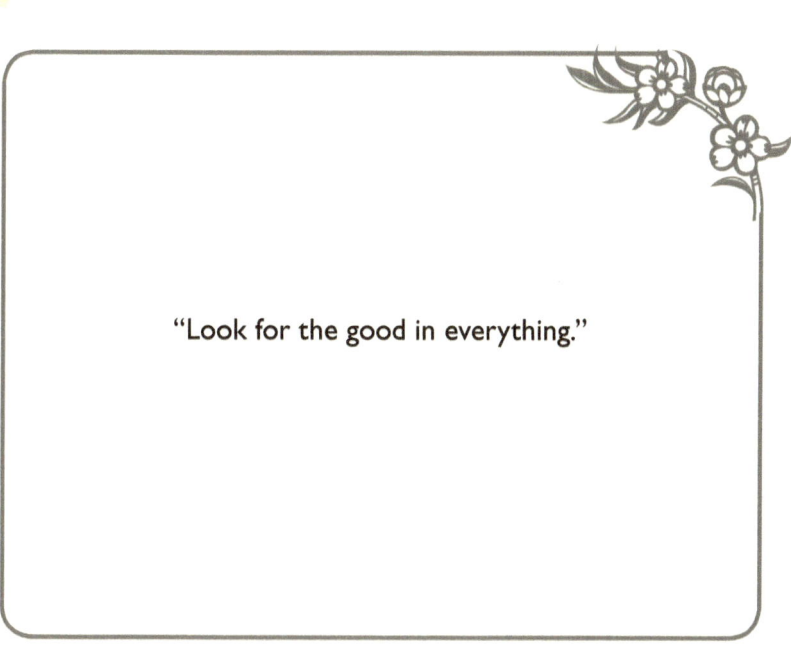

"Look for the good in everything."

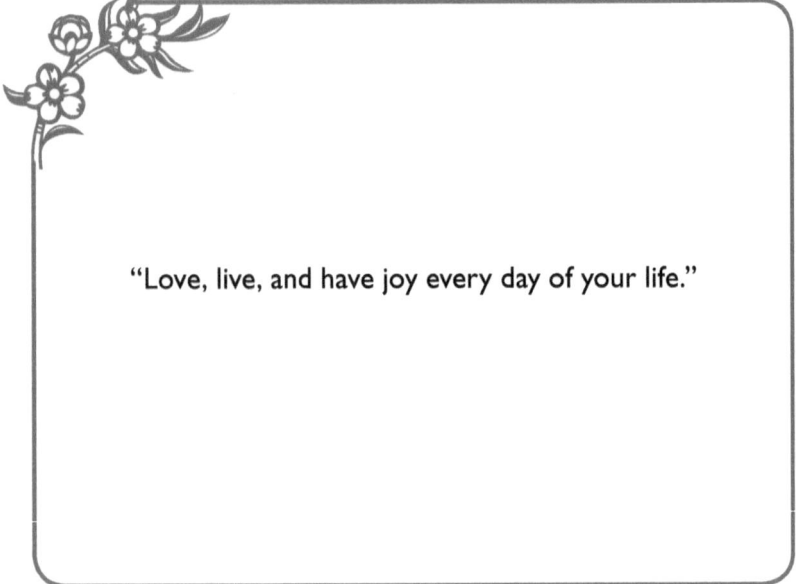

"Love, live, and have joy every day of your life."

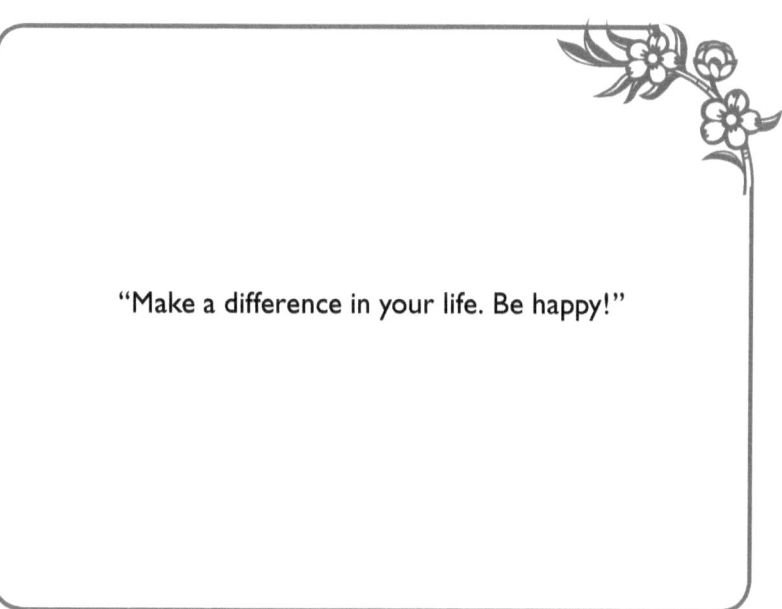

"Make a difference in your life. Be happy!"

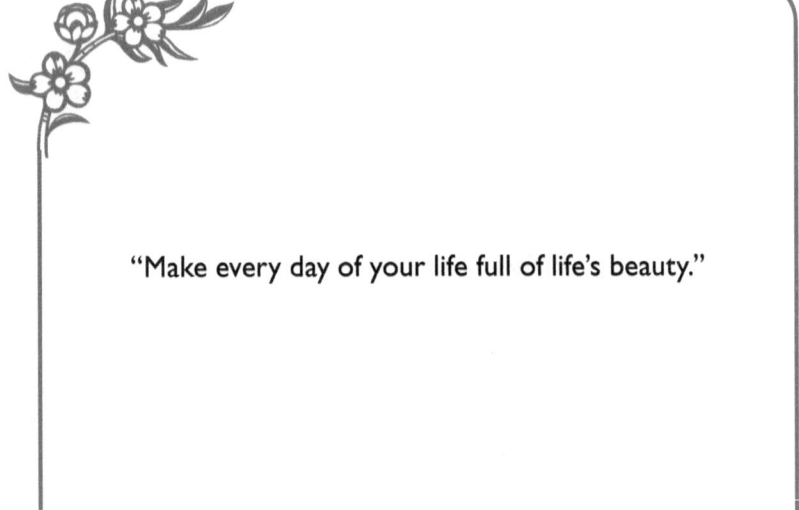

"Make every day of your life full of life's beauty."

"Make food your medicine
and medicine your food."
Hippocrates

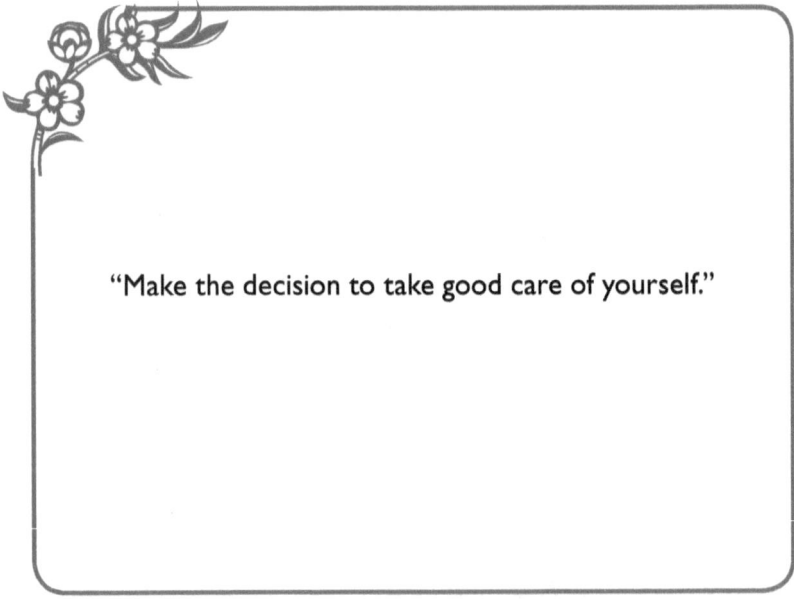

"Make the decision to take good care of yourself."

"Make the difference and
be the difference in life."
Wayne Dyer, MD

"Moderate eating ensures sound
sleep and a clear mind."
Andrew Weil, MD

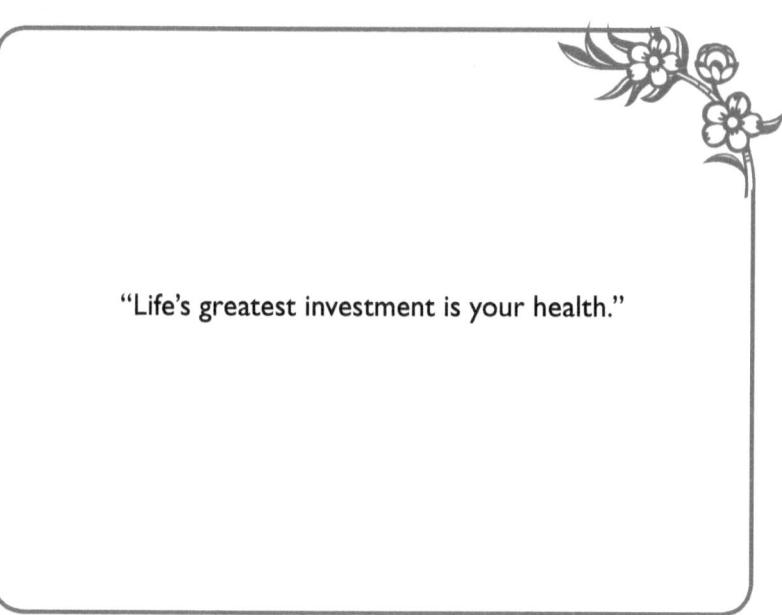

"Life's greatest investment is your health."

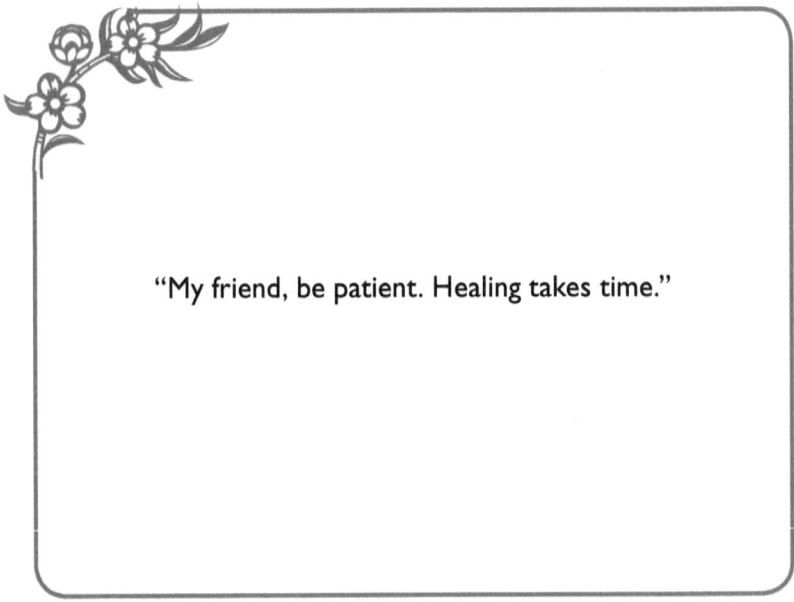

"My friend, be patient. Healing takes time."

"Never give up hope. Paint in your mind
bright and happy expectations."

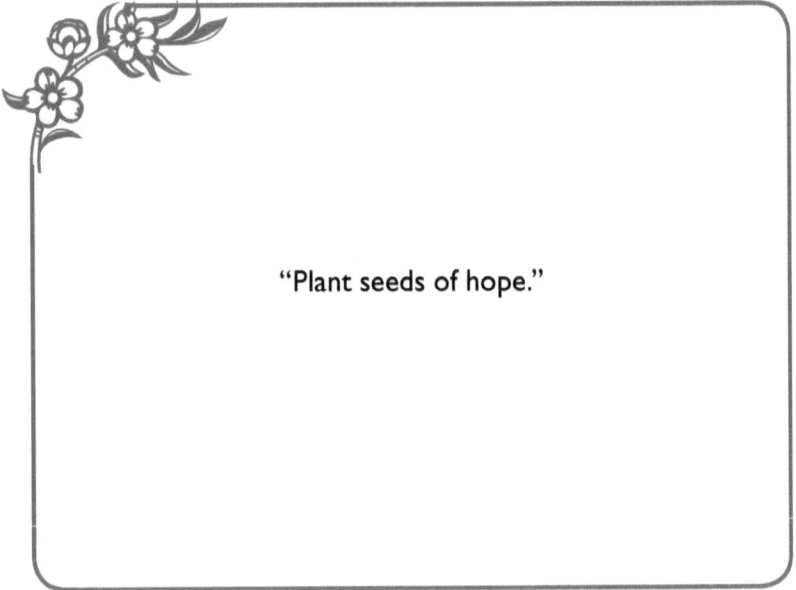

"Plant seeds of hope."

"Positive words can strengthen
your immune system."

"Preserve your health with little stress,
good sleep, and a joyful heart."

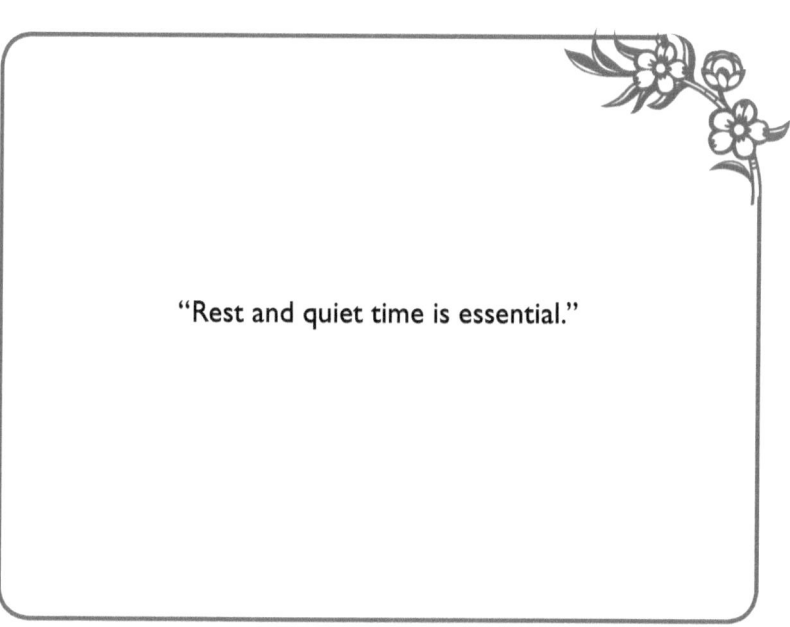

"Rest and quiet time is essential."

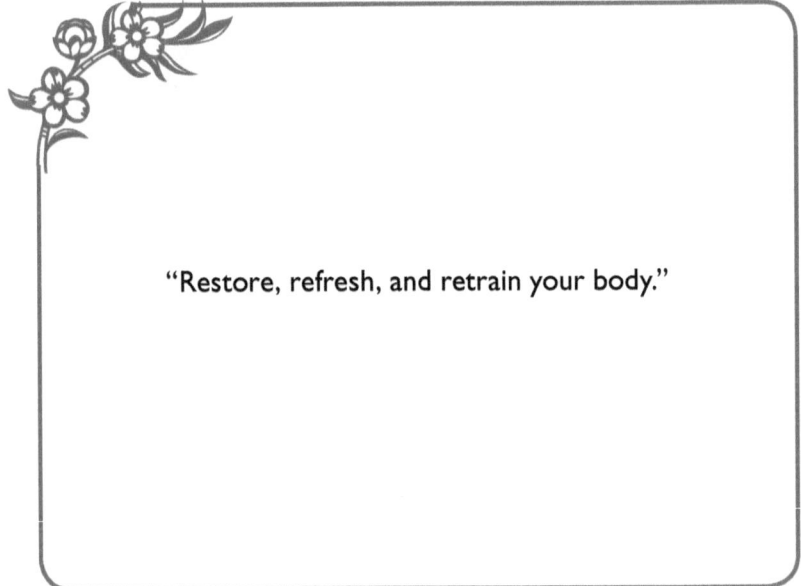

"Restore, refresh, and retrain your body."

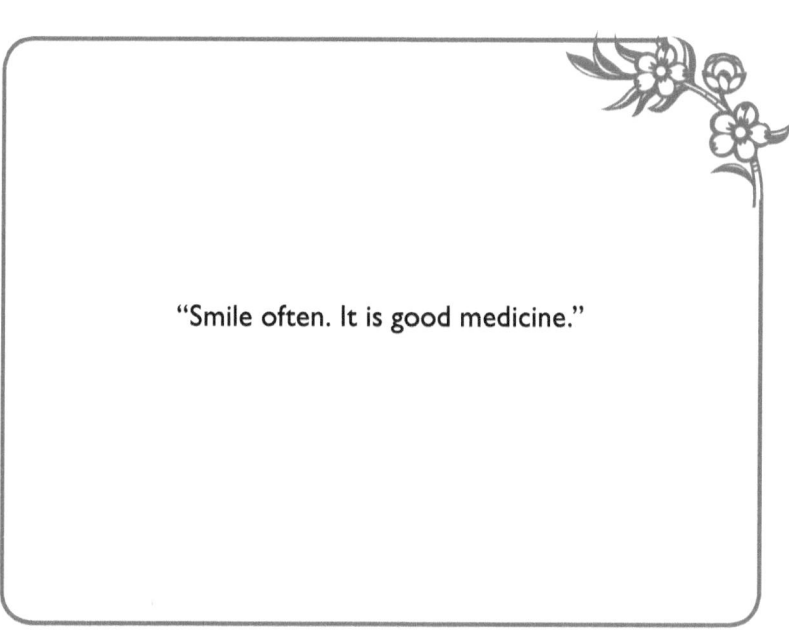

"Smile often. It is good medicine."

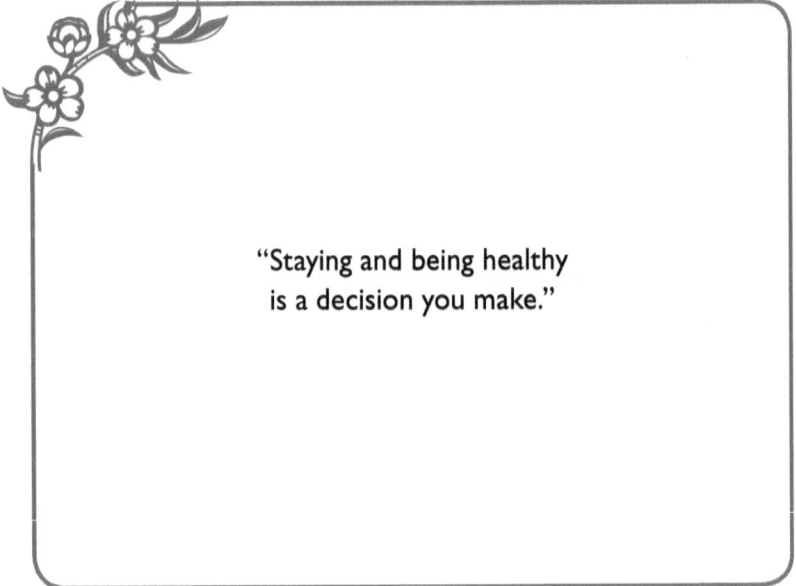

"Staying and being healthy
is a decision you make."

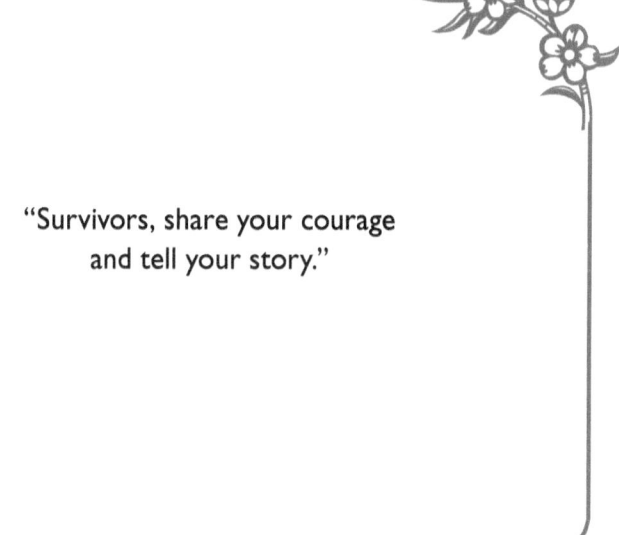

"Survivors, share your courage
and tell your story."

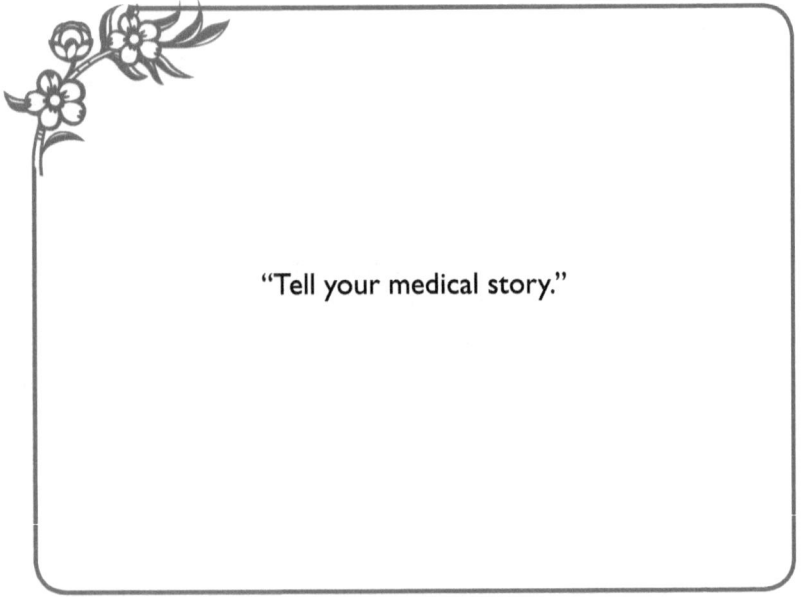

"Tell your medical story."

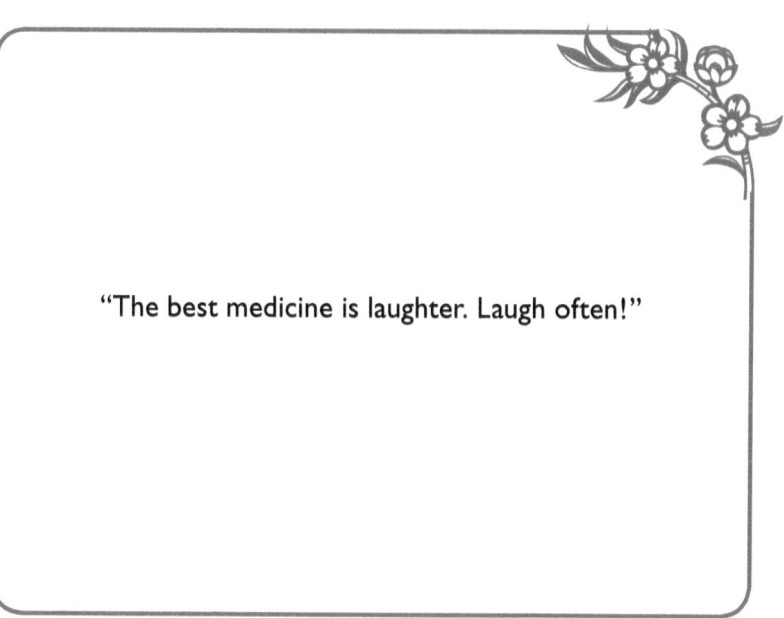

"The best medicine is laughter. Laugh often!"

"The good news is that today
you can choose to be well."

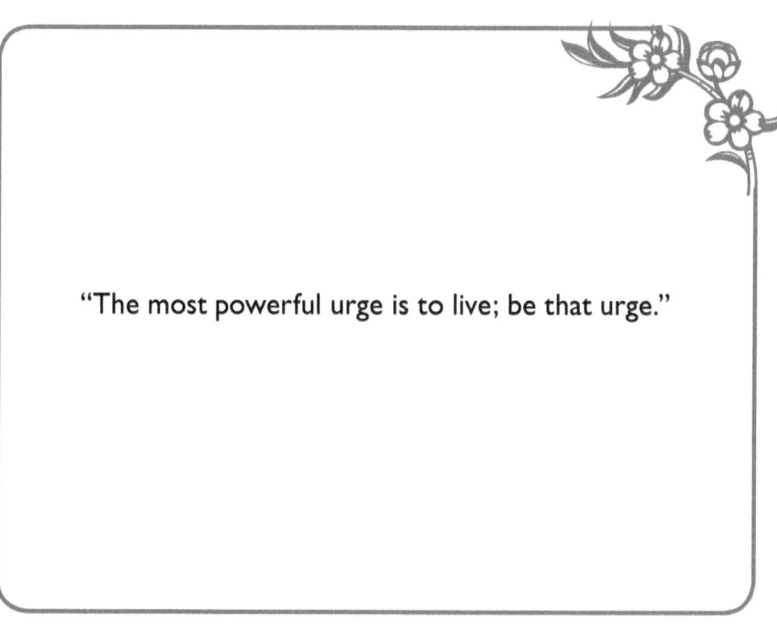

"The most powerful urge is to live; be that urge."

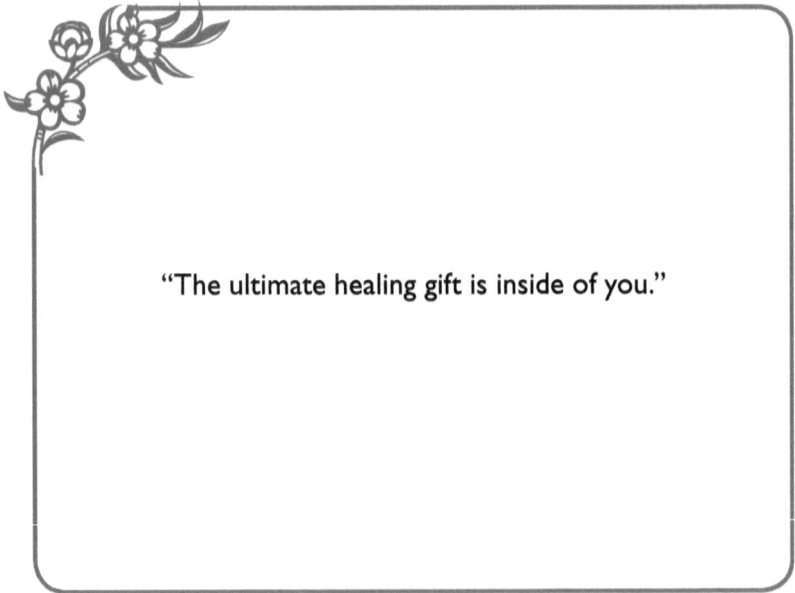

"The ultimate healing gift is inside of you."

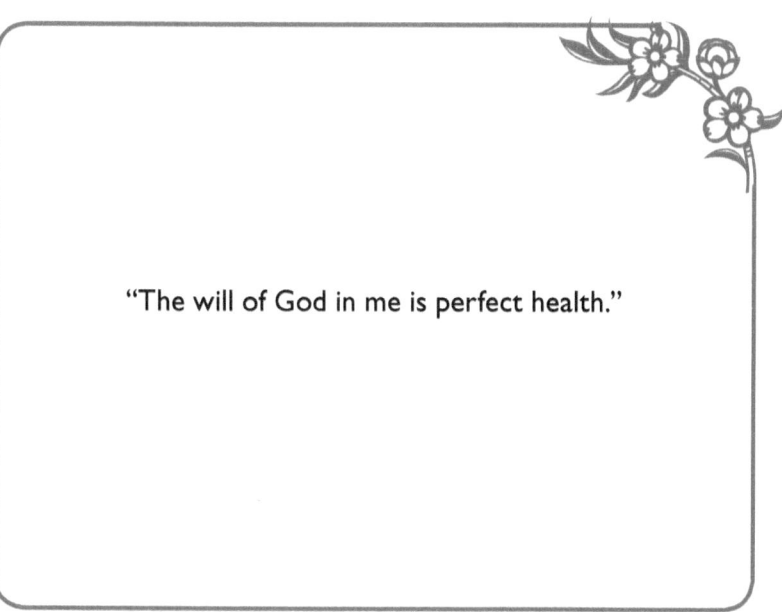

"The will of God in me is perfect health."

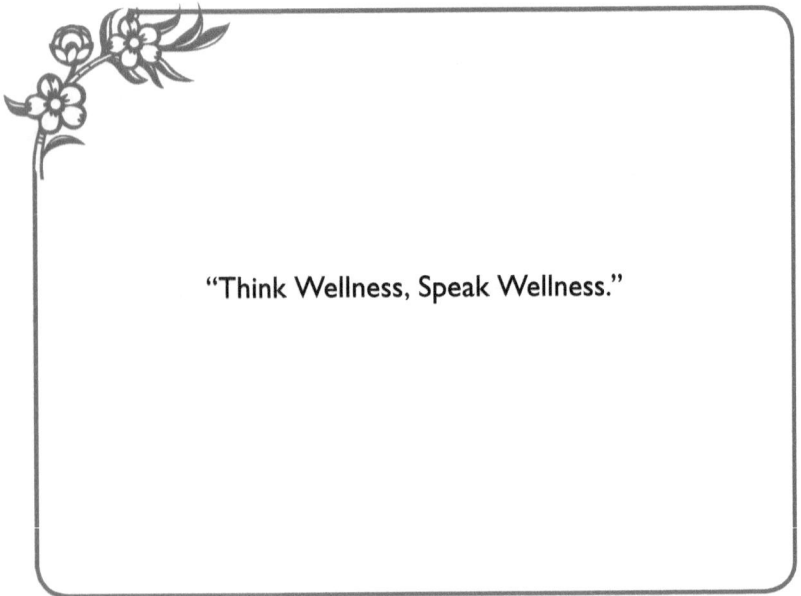

"Think Wellness, Speak Wellness."

"Through lack of self-control, many have died. Abstemious from harmful substances and toxic substances prolongs man's life."
King James Bible

"To your good health, clean air, balanced diet,
exercise, rest, sunshine, and water."

"Today, I will do my best in being healthier than yesterday."

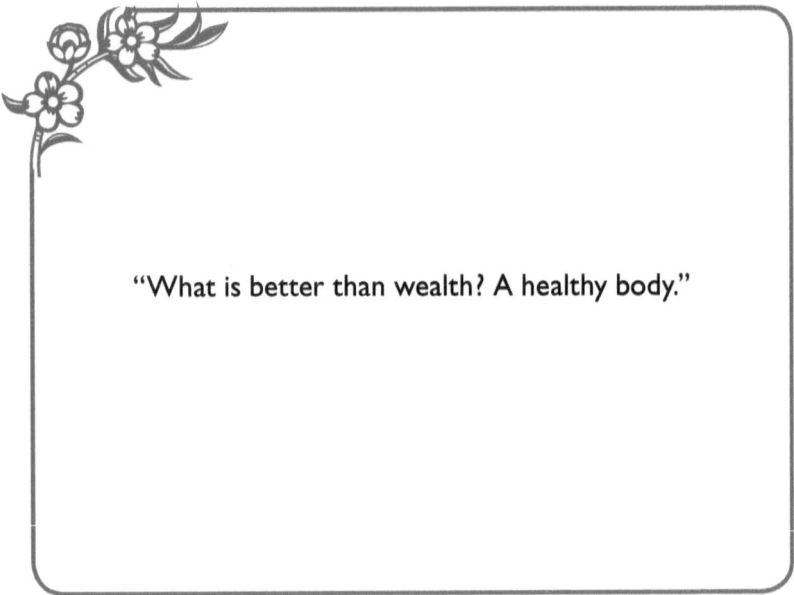

"What is better than wealth? A healthy body."

"Whenever the world frowns at me,
I give back a big smile."

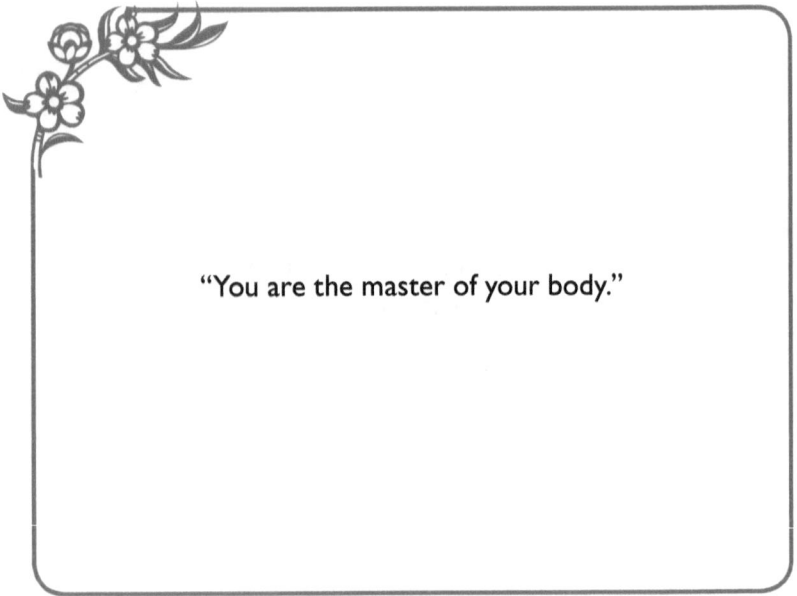

"You are the master of your body."

The following pages will assist you with organizing your personal medical information: doctor's appointments, clinic appointments, medications, blood type, and other pertinent information.

Use it to follow-up and store medical information that may empower you further as you journey through the medical establishment.

ALLERGIES

Allergies are disorders of the immune system. A person's immune system reacts to substances in the environment such as mold, pollen, animal fur, and insect bites. Reactions can be very common as well as serious. Symptoms may include, but are not limited to itching, hives, swelling, trouble breathing, or anaphylaxis. The causes of allergic reactions can also come from foods such as seafood, fruits, and nuts.

Allergies can make life very difficult. Make sure you know what your allergies are. It can make a difference between life and death for many.

Most allergies respond to antihistamine and epinephrine. Being ready and prepared to treat allergic reactions are of great importance. If you need an EpiPen, always have your auto injector with you in case an emergency occurs.

Remember to visit your Primary Care Provider for an evaluation and a referral to a specialist for treatment of allergy symptoms.

List

Allergies / Medications / Date of Occurrence

_____

_____

_____

_____

_____

_____

_____

_____

_____

_____

_____

_____

_____

_____

_____

_____

_____

_____

_____

_____

_____

_____

_____

_____

_____

_____

_____

_____

BIRTH CHART

Congratulations on your new addition to the family. Now it is time to write down important facts about your new baby.

Baby's Name
Birth Marks
Birth date
Birth weight
Father's Name
Mothers' Name
Birth Information
Blood Type
Hospital
Doctor's Name
Parents' Genetic information results (helps people make solid decision about their future)

BLOOD PRESSURE

Blood pressure is the force of blood pushing against your blood vessels' walls. The heart pumps the blood through the blood vessels to circulate throughout the entire body.

Knowing your blood pressure numbers is important to not only feel better, but for your total health care. High blood pressure can affect heart, kidney, and cardiovascular health. Low blood pressure, known as hypotension, occurs when blood pressure falls below 90/60. Low blood pressure is often not serious and can be the result of a minor issue. However, some may experience low blood pressure because of some underlying condition. If you experience any low blood pressure symptoms, it is important to consult a doctor to determine their cause.

Many physiological factors that can affect your blood pressure readings: diet, obesity, drugs, smoking, stress, alcohol, and genetic markings.

Keep in mind that your blood pressure may change slightly with exercise, losing weight, stress, or sleep patterns. The American Heart Association indicates that the normal blood pressure is 120/80 for an adult age 20 or over.

The upper number is your systolic and is where most attention is given. The lower number is the diastolic number.

List your Blood Pressure Numbers and date when taken.

_____

_____

_____

_____

_____

_____

_____

_____

_____

_____

_____

_____

_____

_____

_____

_____

_____

_____

_____

_____

_____

_____

_____

_____

_____

BLOOD TYPE

Know your blood type. It is a classification of blood based on the presence or absence of inherited antigenic substances on the surfaces of red blood cells. These antigens may be proteins.

Blood consists of carbohydrates, glycoproteins, or glycolipids. An adult human has about 4-6 liters of blood circulating in the body. Among other things, blood transports oxygen to various parts of the body. Blood types are generally A, B, AB and O.

Did you know, almost 40% of the population has O blood? Type O blood is the universal blood type and is the only type that other blood types can use.

What is your blood type?

_____

_____

_____

PLAN FOR BURIAL RITES, MEMORIAL, OR SERVICE PLAN

Life and death is simple. We humans make it complicated.

Death is inevitable, it will happen to each and every one of us.

The Wellness Journal recommends that you be prepared. Start a discussion with your family and if you can, inform loved ones of your wishes. Inform them of how you would like to be remembered. Let them know whether you want a memorial service, to be cremated, a traditional funeral, or some other type of service. Also, plan details about how you wish to be dressed, the church for the services, songs, and any special requests you have. Having the conversation and the plan will be of honor and value to your love ones.

Share and begin your information here.

_____

_____

_____

_____

_____

_____

_____

_____

_____

_____

_____

_____

_____

_____

This page is dedicated to two people that I loved and will forever remember, my mother Maria Tereza and Amirah Winslow. They were both diagnosed with cancer and lived for many years, courageous angels that they were.

Cancer is a word that carries so much fear and pain. Very few people can accept the word "cancer" as a positive word due to the uncertainties of this disease. There are many cancers and many cancer treatments. Today, the treatments are improved and people are living longer and enjoying their lives fully. People are learning not to give up the fight. They are full of faith and courage.

When diagnosed with cancer, there will be good days and bad days. Remember that your attitude is what makes life worth living. Be as knowledgeable as possible. Talk to your physician, join groups, talk to family members, and embrace your healing fully. Try to relax often and work with the healthy side of life. Eat well, exercise, laugh, and work on living with less stress.

List your cancer origin / Date of Diagnosis

DAILY DIET INTAKE

Keep a record of your daily intake. Listing what you consume on a daily basis is a way to measure how balanced your diet is. Are you receiving the proper daily nutrients? What nutrients may you need to add or delete from your diet?

Is your diet like a caveman, a Soul food lover, or more like a junk food junkie? You may not have a uniform plan, but there are certain food groups that you eat regularly.

THE WELLNESS JOURNAL RECOMMENDS TO EAT REAL FOODS

Keep a record of your diet / Write it down

_____

_____

_____

_____

_____

_____

_____

_____

_____

_____

_____

_____

_____

_____

_____

_____

_____

DENTAL INFORMATION

Dental care is one of those services that you can't live without. Finding the right dentist is necessary for your ongoing dental hygiene needs.

Having a great dentist makes life sweet and is like having a lifesaver. We all need to visit the dentist from time to time, either to have our teeth cleaned or other dental procedures. It's difficult enough to visit the dentist, so why not find a dental provider that you have confidence in and can trust?

The right dentist will assist with the prevention of tooth decay, root canal therapy, extractions, fillings, crowns, bridges, and full and partial dentures.

You can check for a dentist in your area. Review your plan details. Consistent dental care is essential to your well-being.

The Wellness Journal recommends flossing daily. It will make a difference in keeping the bacteria at bay and will reduce cavities between your teeth.

Name of Dentist / Location / Date of Last Appointment

DIABETES

Diabetes is one of the most serious health conditions in the United States. Millions of people have diabetes all over the world. It is a challenging diagnosis. Diabetes, simply put, is when a large amount of sugar is in the bloodstream. Normally a hormone called insulin balances the sugar, but with the case of diabetes, the hormone is off balance.

There are two types of diabetes, Juvenile diabetes, which is insulin dependent diabetes, and type 2 diabetes. Type 2 accounts for ninety five percent of the cases diagnosed. Once diagnosed with diabetes, you can control it. You will need to work on your blood sugar, blood pressure, weight, cholesterol, and stress. This may possibly move you towards not needing any medication.

A few symptoms of diabetes can be being thirsty often, constant urination, a tickling of hand and feet, and sleep issues.

Type of diabetes / When diagnosed / What are your numbers

_____

_____

_____

_____

_____

_____

_____

_____

_____

_____

_____

EMERGENCY CALLS

In case of emergency, the need to contact someone to assist and support you is of great importance. The Wellness Journal recommends having emergency numbers that you update frequently. They should include family members, primary care doctor, dental emergency, and other numbers that are important to you.

Remember, someone in your life cares about you and your well-being, so keep the numbers posted and updated.

List Name / Phone Number

_____

_____

_____

_____

_____

_____

_____

_____

_____

_____

_____

_____

_____

_____

_____

_____

_____

EMERGENCY ROOM VISITS

It is important to keep in mind that emergency rooms are for saving lives, not for treatment on a "first come, first served" basis. The patient with the most critical condition is the priority. Emergency rooms around the country are open twenty-four hours for your immediate situation or crisis.

List all emergency room visits you have had in the past few years. List where, when, and why you were there.

Date seen / Hospital Emergency

_____

_____

_____

_____

_____

_____

_____

_____

_____

_____

_____

_____

_____

_____

_____

_____

_____

END OF LIFE CARE

End of life care takes planning. This is something you need to discuss with family members. It is not an easy decision to make, but it will be extremely valuable to family members to know what your decision for your end of life plans are. It is important to have an honest discussion with the people in your life who will support you with your decision.

End of life care discussions should also include the support of physical, mental, and emotional support providers.

When you decide on the level of care, ask your treatment team about the advance directives. Advance directives are legal documents that re-cord a person's wishes for end of life care, such as whether to resuscitate or not. Again, this is your decision along with your loved ones.

Other options are Hospice Care or other facilities that provide in-home or group home care and support. Ask your health provider for additional service information within your community.

Begin the decision here. Write down the information and share with family members.

_____

_____

_____

_____

_____

_____

_____

_____

_____

_____

_____

_____

_____

_____

_____

_____

_____

_____

_____

_____

_____

_____

_____

_____

_____

_____

_____

_____

_____

EYE HEALTH

When choosing an eye care professional, remember to have a vision examination on a regular basis. Seek an optometrist for normal vision procedures and yearly checkups. If you wear glasses, take them along with you during your vision check-up.

An ophthalmologist is a medical doctor specializing in eye conditions and diseases. They can handle surgeries of the eye and other eye complications.

Eye Care Professionals / Location / Date

_____

_____

_____

_____

_____

_____

_____

_____

_____

_____

_____

_____

_____

_____

_____

_____

_____

_____

FAMILY HISTORY

Knowing your family medical history tree is very important. The information concerning certain medical diseases, illnesses, or medical issues is of value to you and your family.

The genetic makeup of certain diseases begins with a carrier within the family. Therefore, it is important to ask, explore, and research your family medical history.

The Wellness Journal recommends having a discussion with extended family members concerning past and present medical diseases. Make it a point to keep a record of the information concerning family medical history such as heart disease, diabetes, high blood pressure, cancer, multiple sclerosis, thyroid disease, and other medical issues.

Start here to list your family's medical information.

Mother

_____

_____

_____

Father

_____

_____

_____

Grandparents

_____

_____

_____

Aunts

_____

_____

_____

Uncles

_____

_____

_____

Cousins

_____

_____

_____

Other family members

_____

_____

_____

FOOT CARE

Podiatry care is a specialized profession for the care of the foot. The podiatrist receives training in diagnosing foot and ankle conditions. He or she can examine these areas and treat all types of foot aliments such as ankle sprains, bunions, hammertoes, corns, calluses, etc.

List Name of Podiatrist / Location / Date seen

_____

_____

_____

_____

_____

_____

_____

_____

_____

_____

_____

_____

_____

_____

_____

_____

_____

_____

_____

_____

_____

GRATEFULLNESS

Being grateful is one of the most important attributes in life.

The challenges we experience are what makes us human.

Being Grateful

_____

_____

_____

_____

_____

_____

_____

_____

_____

_____

_____

_____

_____

_____

_____

_____

_____

_____

_____

_____

_____

_____

HOME HEALTH SUPPLIES

List your home health supply products and location.

The use of home health equipment and supplies are a necessary service for those that are in need of assistance. Keep in mind that decisions about selection of equipment (beds, wheelchair, commodes, bedpans, incontinence care products, etc.) must be based on the suitability of the patient's home care needs, environment, and lifestyle. Your home health care team or the hospital will be able to assist you with the selections.

List Supplier / Location / Date of Placement

_____

_____

_____

_____

_____

_____

_____

_____

_____

_____

_____

_____

_____

_____

_____

_____

_____

INSURANCE INFORMATION

Keeping a record of your insurance, complete with identification number, is important when entering a medical facility for services. To have all your vital medical information written down in one place will be a relief in times of an emergency. Whether it is Medicare, Medicaid, or private insurance, keep all of the information updated. At times, finding the card in our personal belongings can be a challenge, especially if you leave things to file for later.

The Wellness Journal will be easy to locate and will contain all of your vital information needed when you visit the doctor. Therefore, write down the information as soon as you secure a new card or a new identification number.

Name of Insurance / Identification Number

_____

_____

_____

_____

_____

_____

_____

_____

_____

_____

_____

_____

_____

IMMUNIZATION

Immunization or vaccination can help protect us from various infections, diseases, and viruses within communities. Shots may be of assistance to you and your family for various illnesses such as whooping cough, shingles, pneumonia, flu, and chicken pox. Keep an updated vaccination record.

Travel vaccinations to some countries are mandatory. Make sure that you are advised for any vaccinations before you embark on your trip.

Update your immunizations
Date   Vaccine
Where
Ex: 01/09/1999   **Yellow fever**
loyal clinic

_____

_____

_____

_____

_____

_____

_____

_____

_____

_____

_____

_____

_____

_____

LABORATORY REPORTS

Your laboratory information is important to keep, maintain, and record.

It is your personal data. Medical records can include your complete blood count, (CBC), thyroid panel, cancer screening, diabetes screening, genetic testing, and others. Keeping a record of your laboratory reports will assist with your medical history.

Type of Test / Date of Test / Results

_____

_____

_____

_____

_____

_____

_____

_____

_____

_____

_____

_____

_____

_____

_____

_____

_____

_____

_____

_____

MEDICAL TESTS

Post your present and past medical tests below. Remember that something that might be insignificant now could be of value later as part of your medical history. List all medical tests such as diabetes screening, sickle cell screening, sonogram, mammogram, prostate, fibromyalgia, colonoscopy, gynecology procedures, biopsy, and other tests.

**Note: Type of Medical Tests / Date / Results
example: Sonogram / 01-01-2000 / Normal**

_____

_____

_____

_____

_____

_____

_____

_____

_____

_____

_____

_____

_____

_____

_____

_____

_____

_____

_____

_____

MEDICATIONS

Fifty percent of Americans are taking at least one prescription drug per day. Medication therapy is a fact of life for millions of Americans of all ages, growth, and development. However, it is advisable to be knowledgeable. Know the facts about your medications.

Many patients are receiving multiple prescriptions of varying strengths that may cause severe reactions when combined with other prescriptions. Know the facts about your medication.

The Wellness Journal recommends knowing your prescribed medications, the dosage, and any side effects. Keep extra pills in case of an emergency, 7 to 14 days of medication if possible. Make sure to label the medication that is taken daily in your emergency kit and try to keep a copy of a prescription in your wallet for times of a crisis.

List Medications
Date Prescribed / Physician prescribed

_____

_____

_____

_____

_____

_____

_____

_____

_____

_____

MENTAL HEALTH

Mental health is one of the most important health obligations we have in order to be happy and fulfilled. Being in a state of bliss is what we are all striving for, or should strive for in our lifetime. We ask ourselves if we are happy and in a joyful state, or are we facing depression, anxiety, and a feeling of despair. We must find a way of being content and happy as much as possible.

See a professional whenever you feel the need for emotional support, counseling, and/or therapy. The support will stabilize you and help when life seems not to be working. There is nothing to be ashamed or embarrassed about. You shouldn't think that these things should not be happening to you. Help is out there. Use it and reach out to someone that will assist you. They will understand your thoughts and feelings.

Provider   Date

_____
_____
_____
_____
_____
_____
_____
_____
_____
_____
_____
_____
_____
_____

ORTHOPEDIC SURGEON

The services of an orthopedic surgeon is a branch of surgery that extends to foot surgeries, hip replacement, knee replacement, orthopedic trauma, degenerative diseases, hand surgeries, and sport's injuries.

Name of Orthopedic / Date of Surgery

PAIN RECORD

It is important to keep a record of your pain levels. Pain can be due to a wide variety of diseases, disorders, and conditions. Pain is categorized as acute or chronic.

Access to the proper care at the right time and place is what every patient needs. When self-treatment fails (over the counter and other methods), your Primary Care Doctor can refer you to a Pain Specialist.

Write about the pain and the level of intensity. Share this information with your primary care provider.

Pain Record

Area of Pain / Intensity

_____

_____

_____

_____

_____

_____

_____

_____

_____

_____

_____

_____

_____

_____

_____

_____

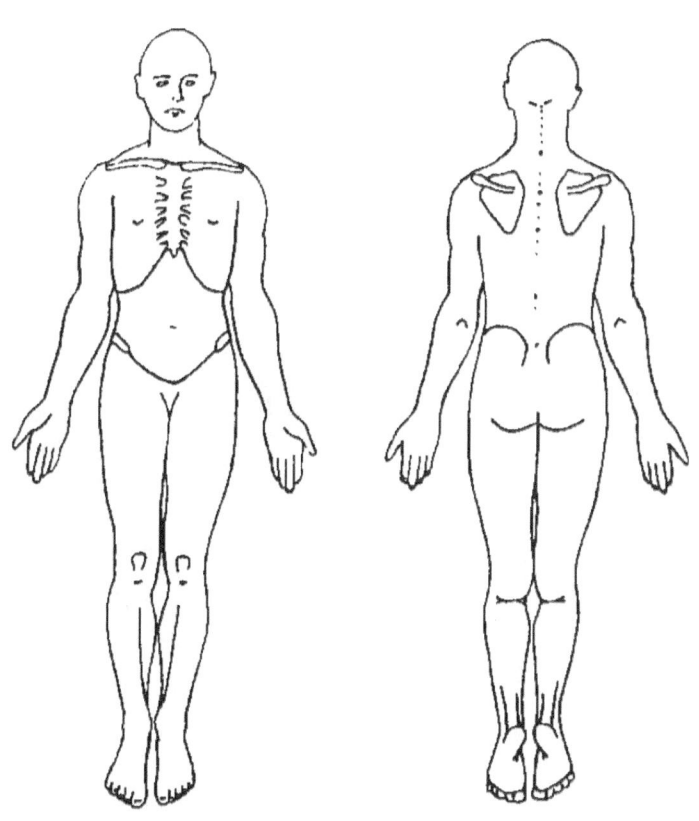

CIRCLE AREA OF PAIN

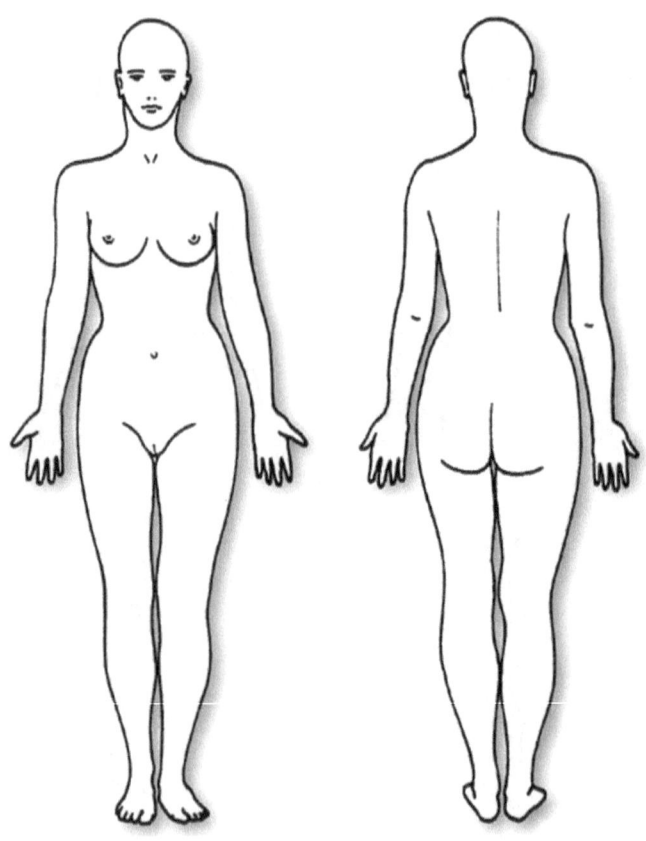

CIRCLE AREA OF PAIN

PALLIATIVE CARE

We know that 6 million people in the United States are in need of palliative care. This is a special care provided to those that are suffering from any serious or chronic illness. The care is provided in one's home in a loving and supportive form by a team of specialized trained professionals: doctors, nurses, social workers, therapists, nutritionists, and others. Palliative care provides to all people regardless of their age group. It supports the care of those who are diagnosed with multiple sclerosis, Parkinson's, dementia, kidney disease, heart disease, and other chronic illness.

Your thoughts on care:

_____

_____

_____

_____

_____

_____

_____

_____

_____

_____

_____

_____

_____

_____

_____

_____

_____

_____

PHARMACY

Be familiar with your local pharmacy. Know the hours of operation and if they keep a reliable stock of your medications. Ask your local pharmacist questions about your medications and share any issues you have. Most pharmacists will answer questions, provide advice, and often recommend certain tips on taking medication properly. They will read the labels on the medications to be sure it's your name and you are receiving what the doctor prescribed.

List below the Pharmacies that best meets your need.

Local Pharmacy / Address / Phone

_____

_____

_____

_____

_____

_____

_____

_____

_____

_____

_____

_____

_____

_____

_____

_____

_____

PHYSICAL EXAMS

List your physical exams. Write down past exams, if you can remember them, as well as the most recent ones. The past exams may give your health providers additional information concerning your health condition. It is of great value to share with your primary care providers your medical history and conditions during your physical exams. This will benefit you and assist your physician with your follow-up care.

Physician Name / Date of exam / Address / Phone Number

_____

_____

_____

_____

_____

_____

_____

_____

_____

_____

_____

_____

_____

_____

_____

_____

_____

_____

PRIMARY CARE PROVIDER

When choosing a Primary Care Provider remembers to choose wisely. A PCP is responsible for your entire health. This is your first contact when seeking care in a medical setting. The Primary Care Provider will collaborate and refer you when and if necessary to other providers. Your Primary Care Provider will educate you concerning your entire care.

List Primary Care Provider

Name: _____

Address: _____

Seen: _____

Note

_____

_____

_____

Name: _____

Address: _____

Seen: _____

Note

_____

_____

_____

Name: _____

Address: _____

Seen: _____

Note

_____

_____

_____

Name: _____
Address: _____
Seen: _____
Note

_____
_____
_____

Name: _____
Address: _____
Seen: _____
Note

_____
_____
_____

RESOURCES

There are many resources within your community offering various services for your support, self-improvement, and available health benefits. Locate and enroll with an agency or support group pertaining to your particular illness/disease. The various agencies will provide updated research, information, and support.

Resources are available through American Cancer Society, Multiple Sclerosis, Diabetes Association, American Heart Association, Meals on Wheels and Food and Friends to name a few.

List

Name of Agency / Location / Phone

_____

_____

_____

_____

_____

_____

_____

_____

_____

_____

_____

_____

_____

_____

_____

_____

_____

NURSING HOME CARE & HOME HEALTH CARE

A skilled nursing home is normally the highest level of care for older adults and those who are in need of skilled care outside of a hospital setting.

As we age, the possibility of nursing care may be a decision to arise in the family. Therefore, it is of great importance to be knowledgeable to what the options are in your area. Your health care team or social worker can assist with locating the best option for your care or for your loved ones.

List Nursing Care Facilities

Name / Address

_____

_____

_____

_____

_____

_____

_____

_____

_____

_____

_____

_____

_____

_____

_____

_____

SLEEP APNEA

Sleep apnea can be a serious condition if not treated properly. It occurs when your sleep is interrupted by the way you breathe. Your breath is actually pausing between 10 to 20 seconds. This can occur up to hundreds times a night, waking you out of your sleep pattern. This might be occurring and you might not be aware of it until a loved one tells that you are snoring irregularly and losing your breath.

List below your sleep patterns: snoring, difficulty breathing, shortness of breath, and other symptoms that are disrupting your sleep.

Sleep Patterns   **Date**

_____

_____

_____

_____

_____

_____

_____

_____

_____

_____

_____

_____

_____

_____

_____

SPECIALISTS

Your Primary Care Provider can make referrals to various specialists, if needed. Services may include the following specialists: Oncology, Endocrinologist, Psychiatry, Radiologist, Allergist, Gynecologists, Cardiologists, Neurologists, Orthopedics, and others.

Remember when given a referral by your Primary Care Provider to take the referral with you on the date of your scheduled appointment. Otherwise, the specialist might not see you.

List Specialist / Date of Service / Location

_____

_____

_____

_____

_____

_____

_____

_____

_____

_____

_____

_____

_____

_____

_____

_____

_____

_____

SUPPLEMENTS

You may be eating well, but your food supply may not be providing you with all of the necessary essential minerals and vitamins that your body needs. Thirty years ago, the soil was nutrient rich and we could get a substantial amount of daily minerals and vitamins from the foods we grew. That is no longer the case. Of course, it is a personal choice in choosing to take vitamins, minerals, and herbs. However, research has proven that supplements will increase your vitality, improve your immune system, provide your cells with what they require to function properly, and support the healing process.

The Wellness Journal recommends that you choose a reputable brand of food supplementation, do your research, look at shelf life, and buy from a market that stocks vitamins regularly. Read your labels and take as directed. You may want to consult with a nutritionist to help identify other supplements you need.

List all Supplements

_____
_____
_____
_____
_____
_____
_____
_____
_____
_____
_____
_____

SURGERIES

Surgery repairs an injury like a broken bone or removes a body part. Various minor or regular surgeries can be done in the doctor's offices.

When scheduling your surgery, ask the following questions: What to expect? How long will it take to recover? Remember to remind the surgery team on the day of surgery about the body part that they will be performing surgery on.

Type of Surgery / Date / Hospital Name

_____

_____

_____

_____

_____

_____

_____

_____

_____

_____

_____

_____

_____

_____

_____

_____

_____

_____

_____

_____

Date of upcoming surgeries

Type of Surgery / Date / Hospital Name

_____

_____

_____

_____

_____

_____

_____

_____

_____

_____

_____

_____

_____

_____

_____

_____

_____

_____

_____

_____

_____

_____

_____

_____

_____

_____

_____

_____

_____

THERAPY

All therapies differ. There is radiation therapy, chemotherapy, physical therapy, and others. When receiving any of these therapies, the best advice is to maintain a strong body. It is the belief that a body that is well nourished will do better over time then one that is not. Maintaining a balanced diet, drinking enough water and fluids, and being stable with a positive outlook on life will help to repair, mend, and build a healthier body. Ask questions. Be inquisitive, especially if you are uncertain of certain drugs or the type of therapy that you are receiving.

List the kind of therapy

Location / Date

_____

_____

_____

_____

_____

_____

_____

_____

_____

_____

_____

_____

_____

_____

_____

_____

THYROID CONDITION/ THYROID DISEASE

Thyroid disease or thyroid issues can be very complex and at times difficult to diagnosis. The thyroid gland is the master gland that controls many systems of the body. Its main function is to produce hormones. When your thyroid is healthy, it is responsible for regulating your energy, keeping you warm, and it controls your immune system. Thyroid conditions can vary, however. The most common are hypothyroidism or hyperthyroidism. Usually a blood test can determine if you are either one of these. The hormone TSH or the measurement of your thyroid function, T3 or T4, will determine the state of your thyroid.

Hypothyroidism is an under active thyroid gland. It may cause your body to respond in a negative state with poor digestion, brain fog, overweight issues, hair loss, and reproductive issues. When your thyroid gland is overactive, hyperthyroidism may cause nervousness, irritability, increased perspiration, thinning of the skin, and your hair can become brittle.

There is so much more to thyroid conditions, so listen to your body and talk to your health provider often. Make sure that if you are having any unusual symptoms, especially the ones listed above, ask your Primary Care Physician for a thyroid panel blood test.

List your TSH, T-4, T-3
List your Medications / Date prescribed

_____

_____

_____

_____

_____

_____

_____

_____

_____

_____

_____

_____

_____

_____

_____

_____

_____

_____

_____

_____

_____

_____

_____

_____

_____

_____

_____

_____

TRANSPLANT INFORMATION

If you are an Organ and Tissue Donor/Recipient:

Transplant Center

_____
_____
_____
_____
_____
_____
_____
_____
_____
_____
_____
_____
_____
_____

Contact Persons

_____
_____
_____
_____
_____
_____
_____
_____

Donor Information

_____

_____

_____

_____

_____

_____

_____

_____

_____

_____

_____

_____

_____

_____

_____

_____

_____

Date the organ was received

_____

_____

_____

_____

_____

_____

_____

_____

_____

_____

_____

_____

Not yet a donor? Sign up and tell a family member or friend

_____

_____

_____

United Network for Organ Sharing UNOS Information, www.unos.com : Phone # 8047824800

Washington Regional Transplant Consortium www.wrtc.com

Notes

WEIGHT LOSS

God gave us this body to embrace with love. We are to take care of it and cherish it. When it becomes impossible to do, we create a body that we are ashamed and embarrassed of.

Take the time to recreate the body of yours with all its bulges, bloating, and weight gain. Thank your body for being home to you and loving you no matter what you feed it, deny it, pierce it, bruise it, or cause it some kind of pain. It's still a beautiful body that takes care of you every day.

Message your body of weight loss, food plan, or future plans. What are your plans to continue building a strong body?

_____

_____

_____

_____

_____

_____

_____

_____

_____

_____

_____

_____

_____

_____

_____

_____

_____

APPENDIX

BE THE MATCH

This Organization has partnered with Stand up to Cancer to provide support in cancer research and encourage more people to become marrow donors.

To learn more, go to be the Match.org or StandUp2Cancer.org

Blood Type

The Rh factor test is a basic blood test that indicates whether you are Rh positive or Rh negative.

RH factor is an inherited trait that refers to a specific protein found on the surface of the blood cells. The red blood cells with the surface antigen are RH positive. Those without the surface antigen are RH negative. The Rh typing factor is important while pregnant, receiving transfusions, and for other medical situations.

End-of-Life Care

The end-of-life care certainly prepares one for life changes or when faced with life ending. A discussion with a family member or loved one to develop a plan can be a difficult discussion, yet it is an important one. It provides the family with a clear direction.

Advance Directives

Advance directives can serve most people; it is not just for seniors. It is easy to see that unexpected things can happen to anyone. Therefore, it would be wise to assign someone who can act as your Durable Power of Attorney if needed. This person can make decisions on your behalf and is aware of your end-of-life decision. This person can be a loved one like a wife, husband, family member, or a trusted friend.

A Living Will

A living will is a legal document that assists the health care provider in following the wishes of the person. Some examples include whether or not to resuscitate, to put the person on a ventilator, the donation of organs, or tissue and pain management. Remember to inform the medical team of your advance directive and living will decisions. Also, remember to keep the documents in a safe place and share a copy with a family member or a trusted friend.

Organ Donation

Deciding to donate your organs is a choice that only you can make. The Wellness Journal recommends that you share your decision with your family and have it in writing. This is a very important process in the transplantation delivery system. You can donate your organ to a living person in need of an organ transplant. This makes you the donor of your organ and the recipient is the person who will receive it. Another way is as a cadaveric organ. This way, the person has decided to donate his/her organs to a research hospital or center.

UNOS

The United Network for Organ Sharing is an organization that educates communities about organ transplantation and is active in the state as well as the national health community. UNOS educates the community about organ transplantation and donors/recipient information. UNOS is a centralized computer network and transplant center. The center is available 24 hours a day, every day of the week for donated organs and to assist in gathering donor information.

For more information, go to: www.unos.com

Obamacare (The Affordable Care Act)

Obamacare requires by law that all American citizens and legal citizens be required to have health insurance.

Obamacare expands the affordability and availability of private and public health insurance to all Americans. The goal of Obamacare is to give more Americans access to affordable, quality health insurance, and to reduce the growth in health care spending in the U.S. There are several positive things that Obamacare provides for Americans. One is that Obamacare provides health insurance for young adults until they are twenty-six years old. A very important issue is preexisting conditions; Obamacare covers conditions that a person has had in the past. Obama-care will not decline coverage if you are a certain gender or have a certain illness.

The Affordable Health Care Act has saved seniors and persons with disabilities thousands of dollars in prescription costs. It is a known fact that the Affordable Care Act has granted seniors a tremendous relief from anxiety over costly medications.

The Affordable Health Care Act supports prevention, care, mammograms, eye screenings, cholesterol tests, and cancer screenings. The Affordable Health Care Act has shown remarkable benefits for many health disparities and needs. Additionally, the Affordable Health Care Act is fully packaged with healthy prevention options. Some examples of these preventative measures are well-woman visits, domestic violence screenings, support for using breastfeeding equipment, maternal care, contraception, mental health services, and devices to help people with injuries, disabilities, or chronic conditions.

Lab tests must be covered 100% as well as pediatric care, dental and vision, prescription drugs, outpatient care, emergency room care, and hospitalizations. All insurance policies are required to provide these services as part of their plan.

Read more about the Affordable Health Act at https://www.healthcare.gov

Thyroid Information

It is estimated that as many as 59 million Americans have a thyroid problem, but the majority of them are not even aware of it. This is why it is important to check your thyroid, especially if you are having issues with weight loss or gain, loss of hair, weak nails, sleep issues, irritability, and if you are always cold. Everyone has a thyroid. Maintaining a healthy thyroid will determine the state of your overall health. Your thyroid is a master hormone located in the neck that rules many body systems. It is responsible for metabolizing food, storing and using energy, controlling weight, as well as supporting brain function, heart function, muscles, sleep function, fertility, hormonal balances, and other organs. A sluggish thyroid has been a common problem seen in the past five years among many patients in the United States. Nutrition, diet, lifestyle, environment and stress are all signifiers of a healthy thyroid. The majority of patients diagnosed in the past year have hypothyroidism. Many people suffer from hypothyroidism (an underactive thyroid), which causes weight gain, hair loss, depression, heavy menstrual flow, thinning eyebrows, infertility, and brittle nails.

It is more likely for women than men to develop thyroid problems. If you feel unusually blue in the year following the birth of your baby or at any time, especially if you have any of the above symptoms, get tested for thyroid problems.

Hyperthyroidism is any condition in which the body has too much thyroid hormone. A few symptoms may include weight loss, nervousness, irritability, perspiration, a racing heart, hand tremors, anxiety, difficulty sleeping, increased bowel movements, fine brittle hair, and muscular weakness—especially in the upper arms and thighs.

Hypothyroidism stems from an underproduction of thyroid hormones. Since your body's energy production requires certain amounts of thyroid hormones, a drop in hormone production leads to lower energy levels. Causes of hypothyroidism include:

- Hashimoto's thyroiditis: In this autoimmune disorder, the body attacks thyroid tissue. The tissue eventually dies and stops producing hormones.
- Removal of the thyroid gland: The thyroid may have been surgically removed or chemically destroyed.
- Exposure to excessive amounts of iodide, mostly from medications.
- Lithium: This drug has also been implicated as a cause of hypothyroidism.

www.thyroid.com

Medications

For some, taking daily medication is no problem. However, planning to have medication on hand in case of an emergency is rarely thought out. What happens to the medication if you leave the house? Does you pack it in your bag or pocketbook? Do you have a supply of medications at home? Where do you go if a serious catastrophe occurs to purchase or obtain the medications? These are some of the concerns that persons in need of their daily dosage of medications should be aware.

The In Case of Emergency Prescription Database (ICERx.org) was launched in June 2007. It is a permanent database with features similar to KatrinaHealth.org. ICERx.org is ready to serve the country in case of future disasters. The website is a collaboration between the American Medical Association, the National Association of Chain Drug Stores, Sure Scripts, and the National Community Pharmacists Association, as well as other healthcare groups. All of these partners are donating their time and resources to keep patients' prescription records safe during an emergency.

Unfortunately, there is no agreement on how patients should prepare their medications for an emergency. The Department of Homeland Security and the American Red Cross agree and recommend that a seven to fourteen-day supply of all your medications be part of your emergency kit. Things to be mindful of: Keep a record of prescriptions in your emergency kit box, write down the medication and the dosages, and make sure you have the box close to you in case of an emergency.

ICERx.org also allows doctors to review your information when authorizing refills or prescribing new drugs during disasters. The database provides drug information and alerts that reduce the likelihood of drug interactions.

www.consumer-health.com/services/com

Note Page

Note page

Note page

Note page

Be happy! <u>Smile</u>, be healthy!
<u>Move</u>, be wise! Be a miracle! <u>Love</u>

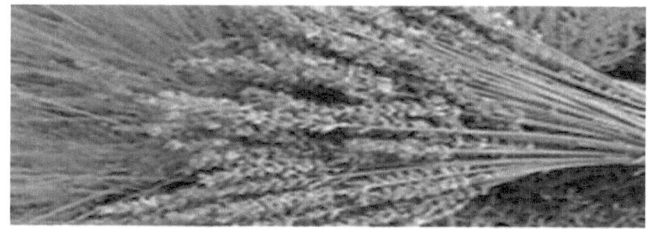